The Dark Side of Stress: How Chronic Strain Weakens the Body

Bachman

0 Summary

Chronic stress exposure and its pathological body-related consequences have been studied for decades. Data consistently support the hypothesis that being exposed to severe and/or long-lasting stressors heightens the risk for developing a mental or a physical disease, which can be summarized as an overall increased vulnerability to adverse health conditions. Notably, the reported stress-related health consequences differ in their characteristics and include physiological states associated with a suppressed immune defense and anti-inflammatory environment (exemplified e.g. by an increased susceptibility to infections), likewise such as states of a pathological overactive immune system (exemplified e.g. by autoimmune diseases).

According to preliminary theories, one pathway of stress exposure entering the body is via the hypothalamus pituitary adrenal (HPA) axis, which is well documented for creating an endocrine stress response. The endocrine stress response adapts the organism to the confrontation with a stressor. Additionally, the immune system provides an immunologic stress response to support the organism's integrity in anticipation of potential physical consequences (e.g. injury). The HPA axis and the immune system are interactive systems which are in reciprocal communication with each other, constantly sending messages created for instance by the HPA axis effector hormone cortisol and by molecules derived from the immune system. The initially health-supporting endocrine and immunologic stress responses are hypothesized to result in health-challenging alterations in the face of severely adverse and/or chronic stressors, which suggests that stress exposure cannot only enter but also *remain in* the body.

In accordance with this theoretical approach, this book aims to contribute to the understanding of potential paths and mechanisms which, experiencing an adverse/chronic stressor (burnout and stressful life events/SLE), leads from a phenomenon of the mind to a phenomenon of the body and opens the gates to various mental and physical diseases in the long term. Stress-related long-term changes at the level of the HPA axis, the immune system, and in the interaction between both systems were hypothesized and tested in relation to hair cortisol concentrations (HCC), peripheral distribution of leukocyte differentials (neutrophils, lymphocytes, and monocytes), and their alterations and interactions in the time frame of one year.

The results of this book are associated with precedent hypotheses and suggest that chronic stress exposure can cause long-term alterations in the HPA axis activation, with the consequence of long-term changes in the amount of available cortisol. Burnout, representing a pre-clinical syndrome caused by chronic work overload, was associated with increased cortisol levels. Importantly, a dose-response effect was indicated by the fact that associations were restricted to severe burnout symptomatology. In contrast, stress exposure due to SLE was not associated with HCC, neither in the cross-sectional nor in the longitudinal design. It can therefore be concluded that characteristics of a stressor such as timing, duration, and/or severity contribute to the endocrine stress response and determine whether long-term alterations at the level of the HPA axis are detectable or not.

Given that chronic stress may cause long-term alterations at level of the HPA axis, this book indicates one pathway of how the experience of adverse events across the whole life-span can contribute to altered immunological defense mechanisms even months or years after stress cessation. Our data provide sound evidence for a long-term stress-related increase of neutrophils in peripheral blood. The distribution of neutrophils was associated with the amount of hair cortisol, which supports the theoretical approach of the HPA axis and immune system working in synergy to adapt the organism to a stress exposure. The long-term (1 year) interactional effect between the HCC and the neutrophil count was mediated by stress exposure insofar that associations reversed under the influence of stress. In conclusion, this book indicates that the experience of stressful events and stress sequences increases disease vulnerability by long-term interactional alterations at the level of the HPA axis and the immune system given that the stressor is persistently appraised as an adverse event.

Neutrophils are important first-line immune cells that participate in the defense and protection of the host. The distribution of neutrophils in peripheral blood provides an estimate for overall immune activation and inflammation. Considering that activated neutrophils are known for the side-effect of tissue damage, a long-term increase in neutrophils may exemplify an initial protective mechanism that turns toxic at a certain dose of stress exposure. An inappropriate increase in neutrophils might foster inflammatory processes and contribute to low-grade systemic inflammation due to stress exposure. Further, neutrophils support thrombotic processes, for instance, through the formation of neutrophil extracellular traps, which can be hypothesized as one explanation for a link between chronic stress exposure and an increased risk for pro-thrombotic diseases (e.g. strokes).

Summarized, this book supports the hypothesis that exposure to a severe/chronic stressor increases the vulnerability to adverse health conditions in the long-run. It further indicates mechanisms that might explain the link between stress and certain diseases, for instance, metabolic, pro-thrombotic, cardiovascular, or autoimmune diseases. Given temporal and interactional effects at the level of the HPA axis and the immune system, stress responses indicating states of suppressed and overshooting immune functions are likewise supported.

1 Preface

In the beginning of the twentieth century Hans Selye described potential pathways as to how stress exposure like an acute non-specific nocuous agent starts a chain of physical events that are independent of the nature of the damaging agent but rather represent a psychological stress reaction which becomes physical (Selye, 1936, 1946, 1950). Further elaborating on his idea, Selye defined the so called *General Adaptation Syndrome (GAS)* as "the sum of all non-specific, systemic reactions of the body which ensue upon long continued exposure to stress" (Selye, 1946, page 119) and appears in three stages: alarm, resistance, and exhaustion (Selye, 1946).

Selye's seminal theory is still relevant today and represents the theoretical basis for a whole string of research questions, including this book. Even if it seems plausible that mind and body are interconnected and inseparably interwoven in their dynamics, it is still partly speculative how these interactions can be measured on a physiological basis. The leading aim of this book is to explore and describe potential pathways by which a phenomenon of the mind, such as experiencing a psychological stressor, is translated into a physiological phenomenon, such as increased vulnerability to physical disease.

McEwen (1998a, 1998b) named an adaptive physiological response to stress experience *allostasis*, which is considered to be the ability to achieve stability through change. In contrast to the term *homeostasis*, which describes the ongoing stability of physiological systems in a way that is essential for survival, *allostasis* is defined as maintaining stability in an environment that requires adaptation and change. Insofar, *allostasis* can be understood as a process that supports *homeostasis* (McEwan & Wingfield, 2003). Indeed, *allostasis* has a price that is named by the term *allostatic load*, which is "the wear and tear on the body and brain resulting from chronic over-reactivity or inactivity of physiological systems that are normally involved in the adaptation to an environmental challenge" (McEwan, 1998b, p. 37).

Allostatic load is expected to result from situations, where stress exposure is frequent, adaptation to frequent stressors is lacking, or where the physiological stress response is prolonged or inadequate (McEwan, 1998a). In later studies, the concept of *allostasis* became more elaborate in regard to the definition of different conditions and consequences. This resulted in the distinction between *allostatic load* and *allostatic overload*, with the use of the term *overload* in case the capacity of the individual to cope with environmental demands exceeds the available resources (McEwan & Wingfield, 2003).

Both the *GAS* and the *allostatic load/overload* theory state that a stressor which is not physical and primarily affects an individual's mind can manifest itself in physiological alterations. Consequently, the way by which the body is affected by a stress experience may not be explainable by the (physical) texture of a stressor per se but represents an adaptive reaction of the body due to the psychological appraisal of the stressful situation. The adaptive reaction is expected to be caused by the perception, interpretation, and anticipation of the stressor and its consequences (Cohen, Kessler, & Gordon, 1995), aiming at protective physiological changes such as an advanced energy diversion or substrate delivery (Sapolsky, Romero, & Munck, 2000).

Even if general adaptation can be viewed as protective and, presumably, provided a survival advantage to our ancestors (Dhabhar, 2002, 2014; Dhabhar & Mcewen, 1997), on the flipside it may be at the price of destabilization and/or depletion of allostatic systems depending on the length, frequency, and intensity of a stress experience (McEwen, 1998a). In terms of McEwan and Wingfield (2003), this price is summarized by the term *allostatic overload* which can be measured as secondary outcomes (e.g. manifested endocrine dysbalance) that are associated with an increased risk for disease.

This book addresses the potential price of adaptation as a consequence of experiencing one of two distinct situations of chronic stress exposure: first, the burnout syndrome (burnout; Maslach, Schaufeli, & Leiter, 2001) and, second, a lifetime exposure to stressful life events

(SLE; Schwarzer & Schulz, 2002). Burnout is considered a stress syndrome, resulting from long-term, work-related stress exposure with the lack of efficient recovery (Van Der Klink & Van Dijk, 2003). It is hypothesized that ongoing work stress requires adaptation to the stress situation, causing physiological alterations that might lead to an *allostatic overload* in case allostatic systems fail to shut-off and recover from the adaptive stress response.

Likewise, it is expected that cumulative lifetime exposure to SLE requires adaptation that might be at the price of an *allostatic overload* if the stress experience outlasts the event in such a way that allostatic systems fail to adequately shut-off the physiological stress response. It is assumed that stress exposure due to SLE is related to different kinds of stressors occurring in different time frames and frequencies. What subsumes stress exposure due to SLE is the characteristic of high intensity and aversive significance. It might be speculated that experiencing an SLE results in an ongoing psychological confrontation with the stressor, independent of the time of its appearance and termination. *Allostatic load/overload* due to SLE might be expected to include an immediate physiological adaptation to a very intense and aversive stress exposure (the event itself) as well as a long-range adaptation to the ongoing psychological confrontation that may outlast the event by months or years. It can further be assumed that due to its high stress intensity, the experience of an SLE might cause a prolonged or inadequate physiological stress response, which likewise bears the risk of an *allostatic load/overload* (McEwan, 1998a).

Both types of stress experiences - chronic work overload and a lifetime experience of SLE - are characterized by the unpredictability of stress onset and cessation. In line with the theory of *allostatic load/overload*, it is particularly important that physiological systems that create an adaptive stress response pass through the phase of recovery. Otherwise, a failed shut-off might cause an *allostatic load/overload* and lead to an increased risk for disease (McEwan, 1998a, 1998b; McEwan & Wingfield, 2003). This might be the case if the stress exposure is lacking a clear and definable termination. Likewise, the *GAS* theory defines continuous stress exposure with a lack of recovery as a potential health-challenging situation that might lead to the stage of exhaustion and manifest itself in non-specific physiological damage (Selye, 1950).

The physiological costs that are hypothesized to result from chronic work overload or the experience of SLE are manifold and include diverse health conditions, e.g., maladaptive inflammatory processes (Toker, Shirom, Shapira, Berliner, & Melamed, 2005; von Känel, Bellingrath, & Kudielka, 2008), thrombotic events (Christensen & Boysen, 2004; Horne et al., 2005), or cardiovascular adversities (Dimsdale, 2008; Golbidi, Frisbee, & Laher, 2015). This book is exploring exclusively the physiological costs regarding the hypothalamic pituitary adrenal (HPA) axis for the assessment of endocrine alterations as well as the peripheral distribution of leukocyte differentials (neutrophils, lymphocytes, monocytes) for the assessment of a general immune activation. Measurable stress-related alterations at the level of the HPA axis and immune cell distribution are considered as *allostatic load* and are hypothesized as leading to *allostatic overload* in the long run, which represents an increased vulnerability to disease (McEwan & Wingfield, 2003).

2 Chronic stress and disease

2.1 <u>Important characteristics of stress exposure</u>

Cohen et al. (1995) define different interacting stages in the experience of a stressful situation which altogether contribute to the adaptive physiological stress response and the 'price' an individual might have to pay for maintaining homeostasis: first, environmental demands define the kind of stress exposure an individual needs to face. In a next stage, these demands have to be appraised by the individual and are weighted in regard of the adaptive capacities. As a consequence, demands are considered benign or perceived as stressful. In case of perceived stress, a negative emotional response results which is considered the next stage. The 'objective' environmental demands and the negative emotional response contribute to the adaptive physiological response (Cohen et al., 1995).

Another classification of stress characteristics which might contribute to the physiological stress response is proposed by Miller, Chen, and Zhou (2007), including the time elapsed since stress onset, the nature of the threat, the core emotions elicited by a stressor, and the controllability of the exposure to it. Both classifications share the assumption that the physiological stress response is not solely mediated by the environmental/textural characteristics of a stressor but by the psychological beliefs or interpretations of the stress experience as well. Importantly, compared with the classification by Cohen et al. (1995), Miller et al. (2007) include the aspect of 'time' as relevant for physiological alterations and *allostatic load/overload*.

The aspect of time is central for another classification of stress exposure. Segerstrom and Miller (2004) discriminate five categories of stress based on temporal attributes: acute time-limited (e.g. laboratory challenges), briefly naturalistic (e.g. academic examination), and chronic (e.g. loneliness) stress exposure, stressful event sequences (e.g. grieving), and distant experiences of stress (e.g. childhood maltreatment).

In line with the *GAS* and *allostatic load/overload* theory (McEwen, 1998a, 1998b; Selye, 1946), all three classifications are based on the idea that each characteristic of a stress experience might contribute to a specific activation of involved physiological systems and might therefore in any way be 'translated' to the body. Additionally, Chrousos (2009) states that a stress experience must exceed the adaptive capacity of involved physiological systems in their effort to maintain *allostasis* to be considered health- threatening, which is likewise expressed by the idea of *allostatic overload* (McEwan & Wingfield, 2003).

Repeated, prolonged, inadequate, or failed adaptive physiological stress responses (McEwen, 1998a), for instance, of the autonomic nervous system (ANS), the HPA axis, the cardiovascular, metabolic, and/or immune system might further precede an overall increased vulnerability to adverse mental and physical health conditions (Cohen et al., 1995).

2.2   <u>The endocrine stress system</u>

The HPA axis represents a highly prominent allostatic system which is known to create an adaptive stress response (Tsigos & Chrousos, 2002). Glucocorticoids (GCs), the effector hormones of the HPA axis, have multiple roles in supporting an individual in the confrontation with a stressor, for instance, by increasing attention, blood flow, and catabolism (Tsigos & Chrousos, 2002).

A stress-triggered activation of the HPA axis is initiated by an increased production of the neuropeptides corticotropin releasing hormone (CRH) and vasopressin (AVP) in the parvocellular neurons of the hypothalamic paraventricular nucleus and an increased secretion of these hormones into the portal circulation (De Kloet, Joëls, & Holsboer, 2005). CRH and AVP reach the anterior pituitary gland, where they stimulate the release of the adrenocorticotropic hormone (ACTH; Ehlert, Gaab, & Heinrichs, 2001). The pituitary hormone ACTH migrates via the peripheral circulation to the adrenal glands, where (among others) the GC hormone cortisol is synthesized and released from the zona fasciculata of the pituitary in response (Miller et al., 2007).

Cortisol is the main effector hormone of the HPA axis and an important regulator of the adaptive endocrine stress response. The stress response and its termination is regulated by a negative feedback loop (Tsigos & Chrousos, 2002) that prevents the organism from overexposure to GCs and long-term catabolic, lipogenic, antireproductive, and immuno-suppressive GC effects (Elenkov & Chrousos, 2006). The circulating cortisol can reach every central and peripheral organ to coordinate brain and body functions through binding with high affinity to mineralocorticoid (MRs) and with low affinity to glucocorticoid (GRs) receptors (De Kloet et al., 2005; Rhen & Cidlowski, 2005).

In acute stress situations, the endocrine stress response is characterized by a considerable increase in cortisol, which has repeatedly been demonstrated by laboratory stress settings (e.g. Trier Social Stress Test, TSST; Kirschbaum, Pirke, & Hellhammer, 1993). An increased availability of cortisol might support the individual in the challenge of facing a stressor, for example, by an adaptive regulation of cardiovascular tone or intermediary metabolism through catabolic actions in liver, muscle, and adipose tissue (Nicolaides, Kyratzi, Lamprokostopoulou, Chrousos, & Charmandari, 2015). The hormone might further promote physical integrity by mediating an adaptive short-term immuno-enhancement in anticipation of potential physical costs resulting from the stress exposure such as injury or infection (Dhabhar, 2014).

In accordance with the nature of an acute stress exposure, the HPA axis can evolve its adaptive stress response in short time frames. The increased release of hypothalamic CRH occurs seconds after the onset of a stress exposure and is followed by the enhanced secretion of ACTH, likewise in only few seconds. Over the course of a few minutes, GC secretion is stimulated by the adrenal cortex, resulting in an increased amount of circulating cortisol (Sapolsky et al., 2000). The continuous incline of cortisol reaches its peak approximately 20 minutes after initial exposure to the stressor (Kudielka, Hellhammer, & Wüst, 2009). In case of stress cessation, the peak of increased cortisol is followed by a steady decline, back to baseline values. Only in case of a failed shut-off and recovery of the adaptive HPA axis stress response, an *allostatic load/overload* (e.g. long-range GC overexposure) is to be expected which might further contribute to an increased vulnerability to adverse health conditions (McEwen, 1998a, 1998b).

2.2.1 *Genomic and non-genomic effects of cortisol*

GC actions are predominately regulated by slow genomic effects, starting approximately one hour after stress exposure (Sapolsky et al., 2000). Additionally to the slow genomic effects, fast non-genomic effects ensure the efficient adaptive response to acute stress exposures. The non-genomic path unfolds its actions within seconds or minutes through membrane-associated/G-protein coupled receptors and second messengers (Rhen & Cidlowski, 2005; Spiga, Walker, Terry, & Lightman, 2014). Fast, non-genomic paths might, for instance, be involved in the GC support of epinephrine and norepinephrine activity under acute stress exposure (Staufenbiel, Penninx, Spijker, Elzinga, & van Rossum, 2013) or in the rapid inhibition of the HPA axis activity after stress cessation (Spiga, et al., 2014).

Cortisol unfolds its action by ligand binding to MRs and GRs. Cortisol binds with higher affinity to MRs, whereas low-affinity GRs are considered as more relevant in situations where endogenous cortisol levels are raised (e.g. during stress exposure). Consequently, GRs might dominate the regulation of a stress response (Pariante & Lightman, 2008; Webster, Tonelli, & Sternberg, 2002). GRs are widespread and distributed throughout the central and the peripheral tissue (O'connor, O'halloran, & Shanahan, 2000). Due to its lipophilic properties, cortisol can enter through the lipid cell membrane via passive diffusion, where the GR is located in the cytoplasm and inactivated by proteins like the heat shock protein 90 (HSP90). Through ligand binding, the GR dissociates from the binding protein and the cortisol/GR

11

complex (C/GR) trans-locates into the nucleus, where it initiates the transcription of genes (Elenkov & Chrousos, 2006; Webster et al., 2002). Two mechanisms within the cell modulate up- or down-regulation of the relevant genes. One is by binding to DNA-sequences, so called GC-response elements (GRE) in the promotor region of GC-responsive genes to switch gene transcription on/off (Barnes, 2010). Another mechanism that seems to mainly occur at lower cortisol levels is characterized by an interaction between the C/GR and other transcription factors (e.g. nuclear factor kappa B, NF-κB, or activator protein 1, AP-1), resulting in an effective suppression of activated genes within the nucleus (Barnes, 2010).

2.2.2 Different stress paradigms in cortisol research

For several decades, associations between stress exposure and an adaptive activation of the HPA axis have been explored for diverse situations of acute and chronic stress exposure (Tsigos & Chrousos, 2002). For instance, HPA axis activation was examined in stress exposures such as repeated parachute jumps (Deinzer, Kirschbaum, Gresele, & Hellhammer, 1997), endurance sport (Skoluda, Dettenborn, Stalder, & Kirschbaum, 2012), standardized laboratory stress settings (e.g. TSST; Kirschaum, et al., 1993), and daily life stressors (e.g. examination stress; Malarkey, Pearl, Demers, Kiecolt-Glaser, & Glaser, 1995). Apart from non-clinically relevant stressors, associations between the HPA axis stress response and pathologic clinical stressors, e.g., due to depression (review: Juruena, Bocharova, Agustini, & Young, 2018), bipolar disorder (review: Murri et al., 2016), anxiety disorders, and/or posttraumatic stress reactions (Steudte-Schmiedgen et al., 2017; Steudte et al., 2013; Steudte, et al., 2011; Wichmann, Kirschbaum, Böhme, & Petrowski, 2017; Wichmann, Kirschbaum, Lorenz, & Petrowski, 2017) have been reported repeatedly. Summarized, it is well-established that the HPA axis adapts the availability of the effector hormone cortisol in regard to acute and chronic clinical and non-clinical stressors, which supports the hypothesis that stress exposure like chronic work overload and the experience of SLE might likewise cause significant alterations in the amount of available cortisol.

2.2.3   Stress-related up and/or down-regulation of cortisol

Long-term stress-related alterations in the activation of the HPA axis have been suggested to result in increased as well as decreased cortisol baseline levels, depending on the kind of stress exposure and/or the time that has elapsed since the (first) confrontation with the stress experience (Miller et al., 2007). It seems reasonable to speculate that in the initial phase of a chronic stress exposure, cortisol is up-regulated to unfold its protective short-term properties like the support of energy reallocation or the improvement of immune defence. Notably, the main characteristic of chronic stress exposure is the indefinite duration and the absence of a recovery phase. With regard to the HPA axis, the absence of a recovery phase is expected to result in chronic over-reactivity of the axis due to a failed shut-off of the stress-specific activation (McEwen, 1998a). The initial up-regulation of the effector hormone cortisol which is expected during the confrontation with an acute stressor (shown e.g. by Booij, Bouma, de Jonge, Ormel, & Oldehinkel, 2013; Deinzer et al., 1997; Kirschbaum et al., 1993; Skoluda et al., 2012), might then lead to a state of chronic *hypercortisolism* in case the stress exposure lacks termination. To prevent the organism from the adverse consequences of chronic *hypercortisolism*, protective counter-regulatory mechanisms can be hypothesized which down-regulate cortisol and/or cortisol effects despite an ongoing stress exposure. Such counter-regulatory mechanisms might explain the controversial meta-analytic results by Miller et al. (2007) that showed either *hyper-* or *hypocortisolism* in relation to chronic stress exposure. If a stress exposure was associated with increased or decreased cortisol levels, mainly determined by the factor of time: the more months had elapsed since the (first) confrontation with the stressor, the lower were the reported cortisol levels (Miller et al., 2007).

Distinctive mechanisms are being discussed that might reverse an initial up-regulation of cortisol into lowered cortisol levels in the long term. For instance, cortisol receptors (GRs and/or MRs) might be down-regulated within the HPA axis or other cortisol target tissues (Fries, Hesse, Hellhammer, & Hellhammer, 2005). Further, biosynthesis or depletion of HPA axis messenger molecules (CRH, ACTH, and/or cortisol) might be reduced or negative feedback sensitivity to GCs increased (Fries et al., 2005). Even if counter-regulatory mechanisms were able to prevent the organism from adverse consequences of chronically raised cortisol levels, a long-term down-regulation of baseline cortisol levels might contribute to increased disease vulnerability in a similar way, for instance, by promoting systemic inflammatory processes (Heim, Ehlert, & Hellhammer, 2000). Effectively, both chronically increased as well as decreased cortisol levels have been suggested to contribute to increased vulnerability to adverse health conditions (reviews: Heim et al., 2000; Pivonello, De Martino, De Leo, Simeoli, & Colao, 2017).

2.2.4 *Hair cortisol concentrations*

The GC hormone cortisol can be measured in different specimens such as saliva, serum, urine, and blood, which share one major shortcoming: they provide single time point measures (Dettenborn et al., 2012) which makes them susceptible to physiological daily fluctuations (Russell, Koren, Rieder, & Van Uum, 2012). The HPA axis is a highly dynamic system, following both circadian and pulsatile ultradian rhythms to provide optimal circumstances for an efficient adaptation to stress experiences and the average daily demands. (Spiga et al., 2014). Consequently, cortisol amplitudes vary significantly throughout the day and interpretations of time point measures are highly restricted or easily flawed by situational factors, such as time of day, nicotine, caffeine, food intake, day of the week, sleep duration, and anticipation of the day ahead (Kudielka et al., 2009; Stalder et al., 2016).

In 2004, a new technique for measuring long-term cortisol levels in relation to stress exposure in humans was introduced by Raul, Cirimele, Ludes, and Kinth (2004), which was able to partly overcome the restrictions and problems of single time point measures: the analysis of hair cortisol concentrations (HCC).

Cortisol is hypothesized to constantly be incorporated into the growing hair by passive diffusion from blood capillaries into hair cells. Therefore, HCC is supposed to reflect a measure of cumulative cortisol secretion over the periods of the hair growth (Stalder & Kirschbaum, 2012). Considering an average hair growth of 1 cm per month (Wennig, 2000), each 1 cm hair segment represents a cumulative marker for circulating free blood cortisol for the month of its growth. Notably, the retrospective review is limited by a steady decline of GCs from proximal to more distal hair segments, called *wash-out effect* (Stalder & Kirschbaum, 2012). The *wash-out effect* restricts valid analyses of HCC to 3 cm, synonymous with three months of cumulative cortisol release. Dettenborn et al. (2012), for instance, analyzed hair strands of 6 cm in length divided into the 3 cm segment most proximal to the scalp and the residual 3 cm segment, finding a significant decline of cortisol between the first and the second segment. Possible explanations for the decline of GCs in older hair segments can be found, for instance, in hair treatment (Stalder et al., 2017) or UV-light radiation (Grass et al., 2016).

Since the seminal publication by Raul and collegues (2004), HCC has become a frequently used, easily obtainable, non-invasive biomarker for the measurement of cortisol in association with stress exposure. Validations of the method are provided on the basis of anomalous endocrine conditions, such as Cushing's syndrome, Addison's disease, hydrocortisone replacement therapy (Stalder & Kirschbaum, 2012; Wester & van Rossum, 2015), metabolic syndrome (Stalder et al., 2013), and pregnancy (Kirschbaum, Tietze, Skoluda, & Dettenborn, 2009). Unlike other matrices (saliva, serum, urine, and blood), HCC proved unsuitable for reflecting acute cortisol levels and acute endocrine stress responses

(Sauvé, Koren, Walsh, Tokmakejian, & Van Uum, 2007), but do represent an ideal marker for the assessment of long-term cortisol alterations due to chronic stress exposure. For instance, HCC were shown to be associated with stress experience due to depression (Dettenborn et al., 2012; Gerber et al., 2013; Herane-Vives et al., 2018; Janssens et al., 2017; Steudte-Schmiedgen et al., 2017; Wei et al., 2015), work stress (Herr et al., 2018; Janssens et al., 2017), and exposure to traumatic events (Hinkelmann et al., 2013; Steudte-Schmiedgen et al., 2015; Steudte, Kolassa, et al., 2011). In addition to associations with adverse mental health conditions, HCC are considered to serve as a marker for an increased risk to adverse physical conditions, for instance, cardiovascular disease (Manenschijn et al., 2013; Pereg et al., 2011) and type 2 diabetes (Rosmond, 2003).

2.3   Leukocytes and their contribution to health

GCs are essential regulators of cell trafficking (Franchimont, Kino, Galon, Meduri, & Chrousos, 2002), for instance, by regulating the peripheral blood flow and apoptosis (Cain & Cidlowski, 2017). As a consequence, GCs might significantly contribute to the amount and distribution of circulating leukocytes. Leukocytes are essential components of an adequate immune defense that constantly circulate between body compartments. By traveling through the blood stream, leukocytes permanently monitor their environment. An adequate *allostatic* cell distribution can be considered the basis for an efficient antigen detection and a rapid, protective immune response (Engler, Bailey, Engler, & Sheridan, 2004).

Leukocytes include *neutrophils,* representing approximately 50% to 60% (Smith, 1994), *lymphocytes* constituting approximately 20% to 30%, and *monocytes* representing around 10% of all blood leukocytes (Auffray, Sieweke, & Geissmann, 2009). Lymphocytes can further be differentiated in T-helper lymphocytes called Th1 cells involved in the cellular (Th1) immune response and T-helper lymphocytes called Th2 cells involved in the humoral (Th2) immune response (Segerstrom & Miller, 2004).

Especially neutrophils and monocytes belong to the first immune cells that migrate to sites of inflammation, which constitutes a first and essential process for immune defense. After they reach their target tissue, they have the potential to differentiate and act as precursors to macrophages and dendritic cells (Kratofil, Kubes, & Deniset, 2017; Scapini & Cassatella, 2014). In case of a local inflammation, chemokines govern neutrophils, lymphocytes, and monocytes to target tissue where the first line immune cells attack pathogens and/or induce a proper immune response. They can further contribute directly to inflammatory processes through the release of pro-inflammatory cytokines (Nathan, 2006; Ueda, Yang, Foster, Kondo, & Kelsoe, 2004; Ziegler-Heitbrock, 2007). For instance, the major type of monocytes, the CD14+ CD16+ subset, has been demonstrated to promote a pro-inflammatory environment. CD14+ CD16+ cells favor the production of pro-inflammatory cytokines in response to toll-like receptor (TLR) ligation (Ziegler-Heitbrock, 2007). Derived cytokines can act in paracrine fashion on the local environment and also in endocrine-like fashion on distant organs to trigger a systemic inflammatory response (Lotz, Vaughan, & Carson, 1988). Neutrophils especially exemplify a paradoxical aspect of leukocyte biology: they are the first line of nonspecific and very efficient defense in fighting bacterial, fungal, and viral infections. Yet, as a consequence of fighting the pathogen by creating a toxic environment, neutrophil activation is accompanied by the side effect of tissue damage and might be involved in the pathology of various inflammatory conditions (Smith, 1994).

2.3.1 *Leukocyte contributions to increased disease vulnerability*

Leukocyte differentials (neutrophils, lymphocytes, and monocytes) have been reported to be essential for a proper stress-related immune response (Dhabhar, Malarkey, Neri, & McEwan, 2012). Consequently they are supposed to play a major role in the stress-related progression of inflammation and disease and are suggested as inexpensive global markers for the assessment of immune activation (Segerstrom & Miller, 2004). Defective leukocyte recruitment and an inappropriate distribution might contribute significantly to an impaired immune defense and represent a key mechanism that links stress exposure to increased vulnerability for adverse health conditions (Romano et al., 1997). For instance, increased circulating neutrophil counts and decreased mononuclear cells (lymphocytes and monocytes) were shown to act as strong predictors for death by myocardial infection, independent of other risk factors, such as age, gender, diabetes, smoking, and hypertension (Horne et al., 2005).

2.3.1.1 Pro-thrombotic properties of neutrophils

Neutrophils in particular might contribute significantly to cardiovascular diseases (CVD) like atherosclerosis, thrombosis, and acute coronary syndrome (Gaul, Stein, & Matter, 2017). Neutrophils provide several mechanisms for the defense against pathogens, including degranulation, phagocytosis, apoptosis, release of reactive oxygen species (ROS), and the formation of neutrophil extracellular traps (NETs; Gaul et al., 2017). NETs emerge by the amalgamation of nucleosomes and proteins derived from intracellular granules (Pfeiler, Stark, Massberg, & Engelmann, 2017). They constitute a protective extracellular tool called immuno-thrombosis aimed at immobilizing circulating bacteria, restricting tissue invasion, and limiting the survival of circulating pathogens. Apart from protective properties, the pro-thrombotic actions of NETs might have deleterious side effects on the blood supply functions of multiple organs, resulting in pathologies like sepsis, tumor metastasis, pulmonary tissue damage, and arterial thrombosis (for overview see Pfeiler et al., 2017). Consequently, increased recruitment and activation of neutrophils and their formation of NETs might contribute to CVD like myocardial infarction or stroke.

2.3.1.2 Neutrophils and interleukin 6

The proportional concentrations of leukocyte differentials differ during an (adaptive) immune response. Neutrophils are supposed to be the first to arrive at sites of inflammation and might therefore dominate in the initial phase of an immune response (Friedl & Weigelin, 2008; Ueda, Kondo, & Kelsoe, 2005). Similarly, mediators of neutrophil adhesion are present early in the course of an inflammatory response (Kaplanski, Marin, Montero-Julian, Mantovani, & Farnarier, 2003). Due to the tissue damaging effects of neutrophils, neutrophil functions must be rapidly downregulated to prevent the organism from inflammatory overshoot and the increased susceptibility to inflammatory disease (Kaplanski et al., 2003; Smith, 1994). The pro-inflammatory cytokine interleukin-6 (IL-6) is suggested to act as potent regulator of leukocyte recruitment to sites of inflammation (Romano et al., 1997). IL-6 might further trigger a shift from neutrophil to monocyte recruitment by locally produced chemokines, which is hypothesized to be an important mechanism for protecting the organism from neutrophil-associated tissue damage (Kaplanski et al., 2003). IL-6 is rapidly elevated in disease settings and can therefore be hypothesized to contribute to the link between stress exposure and increased disease vulnerability (Hunter & Jones, 2015).

2.4   The interaction between HPA axis and immune system

Human as well as animal data provide strong evidence that exposure to stress can dysregulate the humoral and cellular immune response to pathogens and contribute to the progression and/or deterioration of mental, infectious, and cardiovascular/thrombotic diseases (Austin, Wissmann, & von Känel, 2013; Cohen, Janicki-Deverts, & Miller, 2007; Glaser & Kiecolt-Glaser, 2005; Lagraauw, Kuiper, & Bot, 2015). The HPA axis with its effector hormone cortisol is suggested to be the essential *allostatic* system that regulates and mediates the immunological stress response (Glaser & Kiecolt-Glaser, 2005). Indeed, the HPA axis represents an ideal *allostatic* system that integrates central as well as peripheral information to provide a protective adaptation to stress, including the regulation of immune defense.

Based on central and peripheral components, the HPA axis receives cognitive, emotional, neurosensory, and peripheral somatic signals (Elenkov & Chrousos, 2006) that together might serve for encoding different stages that form the adaptive stress response, including perception of environmental demands, appraisal, and emotional response (Cohen et al., 1995). Together, this information might serve to provide an optimal immune defense in anticipation of potential damage, such as being injured in a fight (Dhabhar, 2014). HPA axis hormones like cortisol and ACTH regulate major immune functions, for instance, cytokine secretion, leukocyte proliferation, and cell trafficking (Cain & Cidlowski, 2017; Elenkov & Chrousos, 2006; Franchimont et al., 2002; Glaser & Kiecolt-Glaser, 2005). It might be speculated that the adaptive responsiveness of the HPA axis, which may be at the price of *allostatic load/overload* in case of ongoing stress exposure, results in changed interactions between the HPA axis and the immune system. Such changed interactions are hypothesized to represent a direct link between stress exposure and deteriorated immune defense, which might result in an overall increased vulnerability to disease (Glaser & Kiecolt-Glaser, 2005).

Comparable to the HPA axis stress response, the immunological stress response is hypothesized to initially protect the individual when facing a stressor. For this reason, immune defense is expected to be enhanced during an acute stress exposure (Dhabhar, 2014). Indeed, the protective properties of an adaptive immune response might change in case of a chronification of the stress exposure. Such a switch from immuno-enhancement toward pathological immuno-suppression was already documented for rodents and is under discussion as transferable to the adaptive immune response of humans (Dhabhar, 2002; Dhabhar & Mcewen, 1997).

Considering certain stress characteristics (chapter 2.1), the factor of 'time' is considered a relevant determinant that defines if GCs provide an enhanced or suppressed immune defense when an individual is exposed to stress. Time defines the duration and timing of a certain stress exposure (Miller et al., 2007) and - in analogy to the HPA axis - can be hypothesized to determine between a protective adaptive response that supports *allostasis* and a health-challenging response at the price of *allostatic load/overload*. At the level of the immune system, *allostasis* might be interpreted as a ideal redistribution of leukocytes under acute stress (e.g. to infected tissue, lymph nodes, or bone marrow). After stress cessation, leukocytes return to their *allostatic* distribution in the bloodstream (discussed in McEwan, 1998a). *Allostatic load/overlaod* may therefore result from any signal that prevents leukocytes to return to their baseline distribution and is hypothesized to cause chronic alterations in the distribution of circulating leukocytes in case of chronic stress exposure.

2.4.1   *Immuno-regulatory properties of GCs*

GCs are potent regulators of immune functions (e.g. inflammatory processes) and are primarily expected to show immuno-suppressive effects (Cain & Cidlowski, 2017). Indeed, controversial results that establish immuno-suppressive as well as immuno-enhancing GC effects suggest a dynamic interaction between stress and immune system in forming the adaptive immune response. GCs can significantly influence various immune cell functions (e.g. cell trafficking, maturation, differentiation, and apoptosis) and the expression of immune-regulating molecules by genomic modulation. During stress exposure, when the availability of GCs is elevated, immune-regulation might be initiated primarily by ligand-binding to the GR (Pariante & Lightman, 2008; Webster et al., 2002). After translocation of the C/GR to the cell nucleus, immuno-suppressive or -enhancing effects can be regulated by up- and/or down-regulation of pro-inflammatory (e.g. IL-1, IL-6, tumor necrosis factor, TNF-α and interferon, IFN-γ) and anti-inflammatory cytokines (e.g. IL-4 and IL-10; Webster et al., 2002). The balance between pro- and anti-inflammatory cytokines might define whether the adaptive immunological response is enhanced or pathologically suppressed. Conversely, pro- and anti-inflammatory cytokines can contribute to the adaptive HPA axis response, for instance, by the activation or inhibition of the GRs through phosphorylation (e.g. activation or inhibition of P38 mitogen-activated kinase; Pace, Hu, & Miller, 2007).

One explanation for the seemingly contradictive suppressive and non-suppressive immune effects of the GCs can be found in their involvement in the shift from Th1 to Th2 immunity (Franchimont et al., 2002). It is hypothesized that GCs selectively suppress Th1 immunity and promote a shift toward Th2-mediated immunity. Th1 and Th2 cells secrete a different pattern of pro- and anti-inflammatory cytokines, and Th1 and Th2 responses are mutually inhibitory (Delves & Roitt, 2000; Elenkov, 2004). By influencing the balance between Th1 and Th2 immunity during the immunological stress response, GCs may be able to significantly contribute to both, pro- and anti-inflammatory processes. GCs are known for Th1-specific suppressive effects, including the down-regulation of pro-inflammatory Th1-cytokines (e.g. IL-12, TNF-α, IFN-γ). Consequently, GCs influence Th2 immunity by supporting the up-regulation of anti-inflammatory Th2-cytokines (e.g. IL-4, IL-10, IL-13; Elenkov, 2004; Elenkov & Chrousos, 1999; Franchimont et al., 2002). The inhibition of IL-12 is discussed as a main inducer of Th1 immunity, which might serve as a major mechanism for explaining GC effects on the switch from Th1 to Th2 immunity (Elenkov & Chrousos, 1999). The cessation or dysregulation of the GC-mediated Th1 and Th2 balance for the benefit of anti-inflammatory cytokines can be hypothesized as resulting in either, pathological up-regulation of anti-inflammatory cytokines, leaving the organism more vulnerable to pathogens and infections (in case of down-regulated levels of GCs and/or GC effects). Or, in case of dissolution of the GC suppressive effects on Th1 cells, excessive up-regulation of pro-inflammatory Th1-cytokines can be speculated, promoting general systemic inflammation. Pathological up-regulation of pro-inflammatory cytokines might trigger tissue damage, followed by additional local inflammation. It might further increase the vulnerability to inflammatory disorders, such as allergies, asthma, and autoimmune diseases (Cain & Cidlowski, 2017).

2.4.2   Possible paths of increased vulnerability to adverse health condition

Based on the immune suppressive and anti-inflammatory properties of GCs, synthetic GCs are potent drugs that are used to treat virtually all forms of inflammatory processes. The use of synthetic GCs exemplifies interactions between HPA axis and immune system that are hypothesized to occur similarly with endogenous GCs. It further provides an inside into potential pathologies in association with excessive GC exposure. Long-term GC treatment, which serves as a model for an inhibited shut-off of HPA axis hyperactivity, for instance, was shown to foster diabetes-like syndrome and hypertension (Perretti & Ahluwalia, 2000) as well as slowed wound repair (Glaser et al., 1999; Kiecolt-Glaser, Marucha, Mercado, Malarkey, & Glaser, 1995). Furthermore, osteoporosis is partly mediated by binding the C/CR to the GRE in the nucleus of osteoblasts, which inhibits the transcription of osteocalcin (Rhen & Cidlowski, 2005). Due to the suppression of growth hormone (GH) release, long- term GC treatment in children is often associated with growth retardation and decreased adult stature (O'connor, O'halloran, & Shanahan, 2000).

A change from an *allostatic* endocrine and immunologic stress response toward *allostatic load/overload* (e.g. pathological dysbalance between pro- and anti-inflammatory cytokines) due to chronic stress exposure can be hypothesized as being regulated by long-term alterations within every single step forming the adaptive stress response. For instance, alterations can occur at GC cell entry, receptor binding, translocation to the nucleus, interaction with cofactors, and/or within the basal process of transcription (Webster et al., 2002) or post-transcription (Barnes, 2010).

Likewise, alterations can be based on single molecules that participate in the modulation of available GCs and immunologic GC effects. For instance, the transport-glycoprotein cortisol binding globulin (CBG) limits the amount of free, unbound cortisol in the circulation (approximately 5% of the total circulating cortisol; Henley & Lightman, 2011). However, CBG can further unfold immunologic effects. In the case of acute stress exposure it works concurrently as acute phase protein which is released by the liver and/or supports the release of anti-inflammatory molecules at sites of inflammation (Henley & Lightman, 2011).

Another factor with the potential of determining the level of cortisol and cortisol effects in the adaptive stress response is the enzyme 11β-hydroxysteroid dehydrogenase (11β-HSD). The enzyme converts biologically active cortisol into the inactive GC cortisone (Tomlinson & Stewart, 2001). 11β-HSD plays an important role in cortisol metabolism and consequently in GC-associated immune-regulation, by controlling the concentration of active GCs available for binding to its receptors (GRs and MRs). The enzyme was shown to be involved in the pathogenesis of abdominal obesity and might directly and indirectly be involved in other common pathological health conditions (Tomlinson & Stewart, 2001).

2.4.2.1   GC resistance

The suppression of anti-inflammatory GC effects might be explained by *glucocorticoid resistance* (GCR). GCR is defined as a general inability of GCs to exert their effects on target tissues (Chrousos, Detera-Wadleigh, & Karl, 1993). GCR can therefore be speculated as participating in a switch from the immuno-enhancing to the immuno-suppressive effects of the GCs, independent of the total amount of circulating GC hormones, such as cortisol (Barnes, 2010). GCR is hypothesized as contributing to inflammatory and immune diseases, for instance, asthma, rheumatoid arthritis, and autoimmune diseases (Barnes & Adcock, 2009). Reported clinical manifestations of GCR include hypertension, fatigue, obesity, and androgen excess with menstrual abnormalities and masculinization in females (Chrousos et al., 1993).

2.5   <u>Section summary</u>

Taken together, the adaptive endocrine and immunologic stress response is constituted by a complex interaction between endocrine stress systems (e.g. HPA axis) and the immune system. A fine-tuned interplay serves to protect the organism's integrity and to promote an adequate adaptation during the exposure to stress. Importantly, not solely body-related characteristics of stress exposure cause and characterize the physiological stress response, but also the mind-based perception, interpretation, and anticipation of the stressor and its consequences (Cohen, et al., 1995). Whether an initially protective physiological stress response results in health-challenging costs (*allostatic load/overload*) or not, is hypothesized as being determined by characteristics of the stress experience itself. Especially 'time' is speculated to be an important characteristic that defines the timing and duration of the stress exposure (Miller et al., 2007), thus influencing the balance between the activity and recovery of *allostatic* systems in adapting to the stress exposure.

Neither the HPA axis nor the immune system and their interacting components react to stress exposure in a static way, rather, they provide mechanisms for a flexible adaptation. Adaptive regulatory (e.g. increased levels of cortisol) and counter-regulatory (e.g. GCR) mechanisms can be expected at every layer of the fine-tuned interplay. Like a puppet on a string, the change of one component can be expected to cause subsequent interacting alterations that might skew *allostatic* integrity and increase the vulnerability for adverse health conditions in the long run.

3 Theoretical models for the intermediation between different categories of stress and immune parameters

The previously reported results represent single and interacting layers of potential pathways by which chronic stress exposure might enter the body and increase the vulnerability for adverse health conditions in the long run. Figure 1, 2, and 3 summarize each individual step in the process outlined in the theory section and map a theoretical interplay between GCs and immune cells that together might serve as explanation for the progression of adverse mental and physical health outcomes associated with chronic stress exposure. The research model represented by Figures 1 to 3 is based on the hypothesis that the duration of a stress exposure (brief, chronic: phase 1, and chronic: later phase 2) significantly defines the adaptive stress response at the level of the HPA axis, which further defines the interaction between the HPA axis and the immune system. Due to the research questions of this book, the distribution of leukocytes is defined as the central marker for an adaptive immune response/activation and is therefore highlighted in the center of the model.

3.1 Adaptive physiological response to brief stress exposure

In line with the theory of *allostatic load/overload*, it is assumed that *allostatic* systems, such as the HPA axis and the immune system, provide optimal physiological circumstances for an individual to face a brief stress exposure (e.g. public speaking). Minutes after confrontation with a stressor, an increased amount of circulating free cortisol is available and able to promote protective cortisol effects, such as enhanced attention, adaptive cardiac output, increased arousal in brain, heart and muscles, and optimized energy delivery (Dickerson & Kemeny, 2004; Tsigos & Chrousos, 2002). The adaptive stress response at the level of the HPA axis is assumed to form a trigger to immune cells (leukocytes) that, as a consequence, redistribute and traffic to compartments involved in immune activation (e.g., lymph nodes, bone marrow; McEwan, 1998a). This adaptive redistribution of leukocytes is considered a key mechanism for an adaptive immune enhancement during a brief stress exposure (Dhabhar & McEwen, 1997).

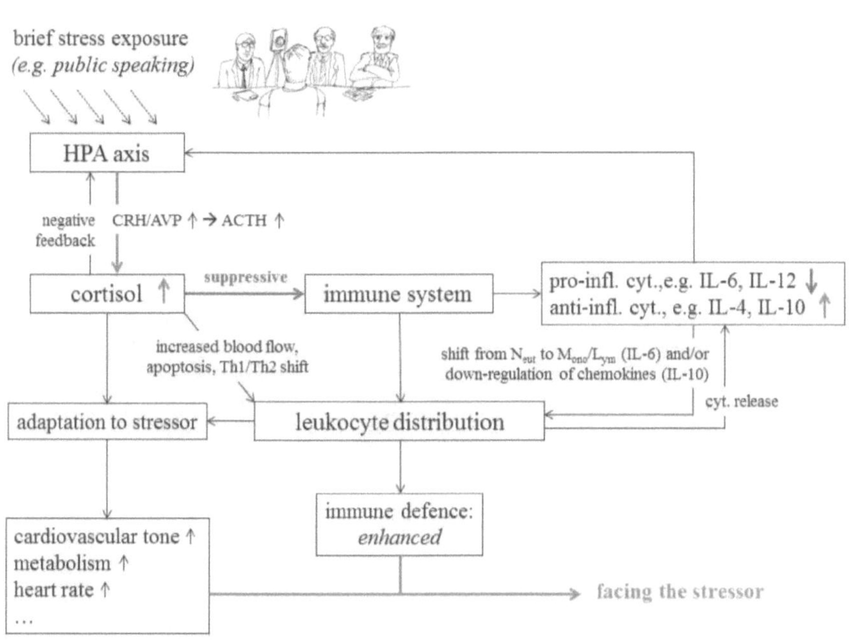

Figure 1. Theoretical pathways and mechanisms for the interaction between the hypothalamus pituitary adrenal (HPA) axis and the immune system for the adaptation to a brief stressor. *Note:* Th1/Th2 shift = shift between cellular (Th1) and humoral (Th2) immune response, CRH = corticotropin -releasing hormone, AVP = vasopressin, ACTH = adrenocorticotropic hormone, pro/anti-infl. cyt. = pro/anti-inflammatory cytokines, N_{eut} = neutrophils, L_{ym} = lymphocytes, M_{ono} = monocytes. (Picture reference: https://en.wikipedia.org/wiki/Trier_social_stress_test)

An adaptive response at the level of the HPA axis and the immune system to a brief stress exposure is considered a non-pathological reaction provided that *allostatic* systems (HPA axis and immune system) can shutoff and recover adequately after stress cessation (McEwan, 1998a). In the research model represented by Figures 1 to 3, (onetime) exposure to a brief stressor is therefore defined as non-pathological stress category, where the adaptive HPA axis and immune response work in optimal synergy to support the individual in facing the stressor.

3.2   Adaptive physiological response to chronic stress exposure

Figures 2 and 3 exemplify two hypothetical states of chronic stress consequences that are considered to differ by the time (timing and duration) of the stress exposure. They therefore represent two theoretically consecutive states and aim to explain heterogeneous results, such as hyper- versus hypo-cortisolism and dampened versus overshooting immune response in association with stress exposure.

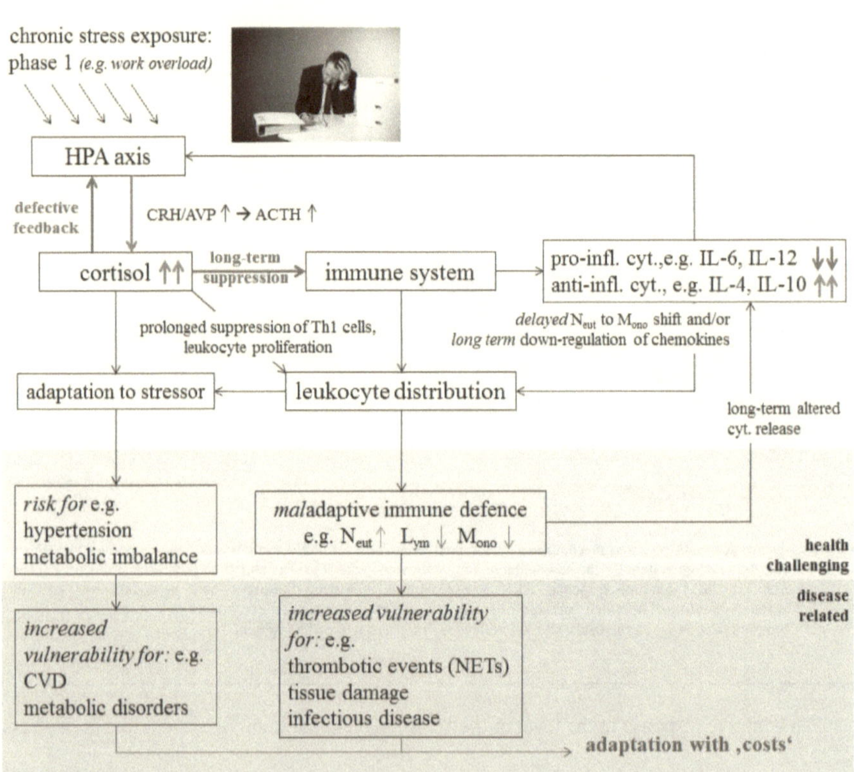

Figure 2. Theoretical pathways and mechanisms for the interaction between hypothalamus pituitary adrenal (HPA) axis, and immune system for the adaptation to a chronic stressor and under the premise that the cortisol levels are chronically elevated. *Note:* Th1 = cellular immune response, CRH = corticotropin releasing hormone, AVP = vasopressin, ACTH = adrenocorticotropic hormone, pro/anti-infl. cyt. = pro/anti-inflammatory cytokines, N_{eut} = neutrophils, L_{ym} = lymphocytes, M_{ono} = monocytes, CVD = cardiovascular disease, NETs = neutrophil extracellular traps, 'costs' = health challenging alterations due to chronic stress exposure (respectively the theory of *allostatic load/overload*; McEwan & Wingfield, 2003).

In the research model of Figure 2 and 3, *allostasis* is suggested to result in an *allostatic load/overload* if the characteristics of a stress exposure prevent *allostatic* systems (HPA axis, immune system) to adequately shut-off the adaptive stress response from returning to their basal activation (McEwan, 1998a). With regard to the HPA axis, chronically elevated as well as blunted cortisol levels have been reported in association with chronic stress exposure (Chapter 2.2.3). It is hypothesized that a chronic increase in cortisol baseline levels might turn into the opposite condition of chronically reduced cortisol levels in case a stress experience is highly extended (e.g. by repetitive trauma; Steudte-Schmiedgen, Kirschbaum, Alexander, & Stalder, 2016). Similarly, meta-analytical results from Miller et al. (2007) show that the time that elapsed between the stress exposure and cortisol assessment explains whether stress exposure is associated with increased or decreased cortisol levels. This conclusion likewise suggests a temporal dynamic of the HPA axis which might explain both conditions, increased as well as decreased cortisol levels, as interpretable as two consecutive states.

Due to the immune-regulatory effects of cortisol, corresponding alterations at the level of the immune system are hypothesized and suggested to explain an altered immune activation due to stress exposure (Glaser & Kiecolt-Glaser, 2005). An excessive and theoretically pathological suppression of immune activation is assumed if cortisol levels are above *allostatic* baseline levels (Figure 2). In contrast, in the case of cortisol levels below *allostatic* baseline levels (Figure 3), the shut-off and recovery from an adaptive immune response might be delayed and/or insufficient (Cain & Cidlowski, 2017). GCs and especially cortisol, for instance, participate in the regulation of leukocyte proliferation (Franchimont et al., 2002). Further, the C/GR can manipulate inflammation-associated genes by encoding cytokines and inflammatory enzymes (Barnes & Adcock, 2009). Both mechanisms exemplify that *allostatic load/overload* at level of the HPA axis corresponds with leukocyte distribution and the ratio between pro-and anti-inflammatory cytokines, which are essential components of immune activation and immune defense (Segerstrom & Miller, 2004). Altered leukocyte distribution and balance between pro- and anti-inflammatory cytokines are further associated with an increased vulnerability to physical disease (e.g. CVD; Horne et al., 2005).

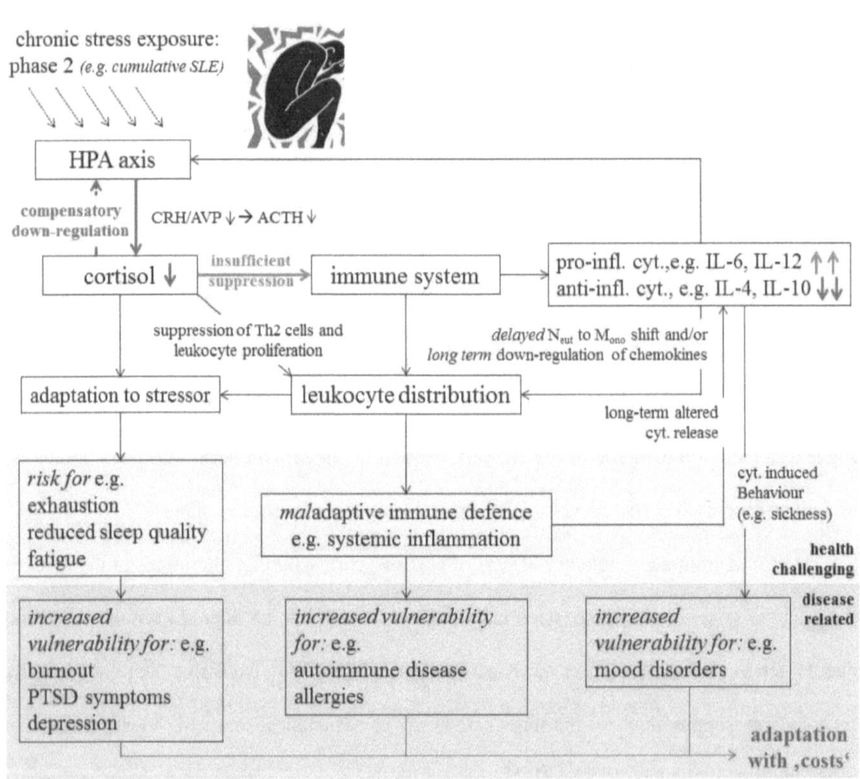

Figure 3. Theoretical pathways and mechanisms for the interaction between the hypothalamus pituitary adrenal (HPA) axis and the immune system for the adaptation to a chronic stressor and under the premise that cortisol levels are chronically blunted. *Note:* Th2 = humoral immune response, CRH = corticotropin releasing hormone, AVP = vasopressin, ACTH = adrenocorticotropic hormone, pro/anti-infl. cyt. = pro/anti-inflammatory cytokines, N_eut = neutrophils, L_ym = lymphocytes, M_ono = monocytes, PTSD = posttraumatic stress disorder, 'costs' = health challenging alterations due to chronic stress exposure (respectively the theory of *allostatic load/overload*; McEwan & Wingfield, 2003). (Picture reference: Lo Cole, www.locole.co.uk)

Besides an increased risk for physical disease, cytokine dysbalance is hypothesized to effect mood and behavior (Baumeister, Russell, Pariante, & Mondelli, 2014; Dantzer, 2009), and foster mood disorders such as major depressive disorder (Otte et al., 2016). Importantly, HPA axis dysregulations have likewise been linked to the pathogenesis of depression

(Baumeister, Lightman, & Pariante, 2016) and depressive symptomatology such as reduced sleep quality (Backhaus, Junghanns, & Hohagen, 2004) and chronic fatigue (Demitrack et al., 1991).

3.3 Unresolved issues in the research of stress-related disease progression

A variety of sound studies supports the link between chronic stress exposure and the progression of diseases. The reported pathologies are diverse and include mental diseases (e.g. depression; Pariante, 2017) as well as physical diseases associated with increased susceptibility to infection (e.g. higher risk for developing a cold; Cohen et al., 2012) or hyper-reactivity to harmless antigens (e.g. atopic dermatitis; Kilpeläinen, Koskenvuo, Helenius, & Terho, 2002). However, the studies differ in their definitions of chronic stress exposure as well as in the underlying tradition of epidemiological, psychological, or biological research (for detailed discussion see Cohen, Gianaros, & Manuck, 2016). Moreover, the majority of study results are cross-sectional and consequently not suitable for predicting increased disease vulnerability in the long term. As a consequence, theoretical models that aim to explain the long-term intermediation between stress and disease must rely on results concluded from heterogeneous study designs that explain specific physiological interactions (e.g. cortisol level and pro-inflammatory cytokines), under specific stress exposure. As a consequence, the long-term interactions between physiological systems that form the adaptive stress response remain highly speculative.

Due to the heterogeneous approaches and designs, Cohen et al. (2016) suggest to structure study results based on levels of a hierarchical stage model. At the top of the stage model are the 'objective' environmental demands individuals are exposed to followed by psychological interpretations (appraisal) that define the emotional response. The 'psychological' stages are followed by the 'biological/behavioral' stages that especially focus on the HPA axis and the immune system. Finally, alterations at the biological/behavioral stages precede the vulnerability to disease, which completes the stage model. Interestingly, most available study results on the associations between stress exposure and disease vulnerability can be allocated to different stages within this model (Cohen et al., 2016), and it can be speculated that study designs as well as results show an increased homogeneity when considering the underlying structures that were addressed.

In the following, the stage model by Cohen et al. (2016) will serve for the discussion of unresolved issues in the research of stress-related disease progression that are addressed in this book, namely the 'temporal' and 'interactional' dynamics of *allostatic* systems. Figure 4 shows the stage model by Cohen et al. (2016) extended by the levels 'temporal dynamics' and 'interactional dynamics'. For the inclusion of the hypothetical endpoint – a certain disease – 'completely developed disease' is added to the model as a final stage.

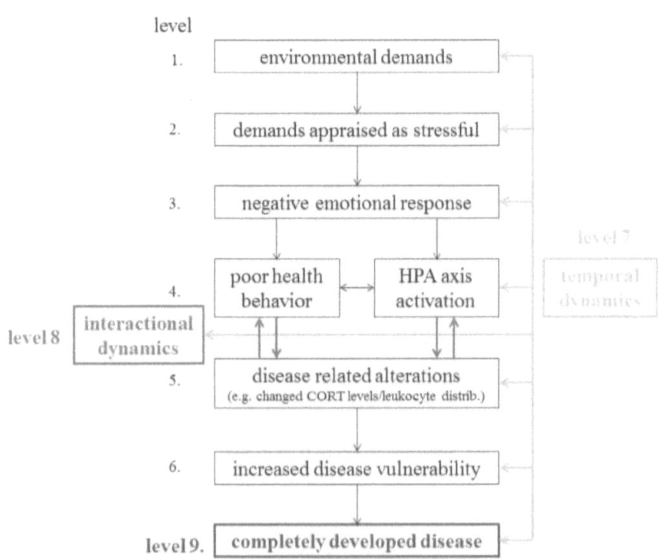

Figure 4. Stage model by Cohen et al. (2016) modified and extended by the author. Levels 7-9 are included with the model and are considered additional stages that highlight unresolved issues in the research of stress-related disease progression.

Miller, Chen, and Cole (2009) suggest considering 'temporal dynamics' of *allostatic* systems when it comes to the exploration of an adaptive physiological stress response. It is hypothesized that temporal dynamics act upon every single stage within the model. At the level of environmental demands, for instance, temporal dynamics discriminate between acute/brief, chronic, and sequential stress exposure (Segerstrom & Miller, 2004), which is considered to influence any further subsequent level. Evidence for the influence of temporal dynamics on the adaptive HPA axis stress response is provided by the meta-analytical results of Miller et al. (2007). Similarly, temporal dynamics are discussed as influencing the adaptive immunological stress response (Dhabhar, 2014).

Additionally, an adaptive physiological stress response might not occur independently within each involved *allostatic* system but by 'interactional dynamics' between all the systems that form the adaptive stress response. There is sound evidence for interactional dynamics between the HPA axis and the immune system (Chapter 2.4). Likewise, it can be speculated that disease -related alterations (level 5) influence health behavior (level 4), for instance, through cytokine-mediated depressive symptomatology (Pariante, 2017).

Due to the limitations of cross-sectional designs which are applicable to the majority of available data, most results concern alterations at one level within the stage model. Disease -related alterations (level 5), for example, have been reported for various immune components, for instance, circulating inflammatory markers (e.g. IL-6, C-reactive protein, CRP, or IL-1; reviews: Hänsel, Hong, Cámara, & Von Kaenel, 2010; Rohleder, 2014; Steptoe, Hamer, & Chida, 2007), dysregulations of pro-and anti-inflammatory molecules (Rohleder, Marin, Ma, & Miller, 2009), and markers for immune efficiency like wound healing (Glaser et al., 1999; Kiecolt-Glaser et al., 1995), or antibody response (Miller et al., 2004). Also, increased disease vulnerability (level 6) was demonstrated by an assessment of the associations between stress and the occurrence of various diseases, like skin disease (Picardi & Abeni, 2001), autoimmune disease (meta-analysis: Porcelli et al., 2016), or cardiovascular disease

(Dimsdale, 2008). Interestingly, studies that address the temporal and interactional dynamics of an adaptive stress response are greatly underrepresented. Likewise underrepresented are human studies that focus on potential stress-related changes in leukocytes, although leukocytes represent the first line of defense against pathogens and are therefore basic parameters for explaining a general, non-specific susceptibility to disease (Segerstrom & Miller, 2004). The number and proportion of leukocytes in the blood further provide important information about the state of activation of the immune system, which has so far been reported mainly in animal studies (Dhabhar, 2002). An adequate distribution of leukocyte differentials in the periphery is not just an indicator of a proper immune defense (Segerstrom & Miller, 2004) but might be interrelated with any further immune parameter as well as with certain disease outcomes (Figure 2 and Figure 3).

3.4 <u>Research questions and aims</u>

The primary objective of this book is the description of potential pathways by which chronic stress exposure affects the body, leading to an overall increased disease vulnerability. Based on the stage model reported by Cohen and colleagues (2016; Figure 4), two different chronic stress paradigms (burnout and SLE) were tested and considered in relation to the proposed hierarchical levels of the stage model. The stage model is aimed to be extended and tested by the dimension 'temporal dynamics' (defined as level 7, Figure 4). Temporal dynamics were operationalized as long-term (one-year) alterations in HPA axis activation (level 4, Figure 4) and in the distribution of leukocyte differentials (level 5, Figure 4). In addition, mutual physiological interactions between cortisol levels and the distribution of leukocyte differentials were tested and considered as 'interactional dynamics' (defined as level 8, Figure 4). For a detailed discussion of potential clinical endpoints (e.g. CVD) of the stage model, 'completely developed disease' (defined as level 9, Figure 4) will be discussed based on cortisol and leukocyte findings.

3.4.1 Aim of Study 1

Study 1 aimed at examining associations between chronic stress exposure and the HPA axis activation. Chronic stress exposure was measured as *burnout*, defined as sustained work-related stress experience, reported for 12 months prior to assessment (Maslach et al., 2001). HPA axis activation was measured on basis of HCC as a cumulative marker of systemic cortisol, considering approximately three months prior to assessment. With regard to the stage model by Cohen and colleagues (2016; Figure 4), bearing level 1 to 4 in mind, with burnout as the representative of environmental demands (level 1). Due to burnout symptomatology (e.g. feeling exhausted from work), the demands have to be appraised as stressful (level 2), causing a negative emotional response (level 3), otherwise would not contribute to the burnout measure. Consequently, burnout, measured as the sum of burnout symptoms over the preceding 12 months, comprises level 1, 2, and 3. The HCC as markers for HPA axis activation represents level 4.

3.4.2 Aim of Study 2

The study design of *Study 2* was primarily aimed at examining the long-term impact of chronic stress exposure on the immune functions. Chronic stress exposure was measured as a lifetime experience of the SLE in regard to the appraisal of their current relevance. The immune functions were measured, based on leukocyte differentials (neutrophils, lymphocytes, monocytes) in peripheral blood. Considering the stage model, the SLE represent environmental demands (level 1). Level 2 and level 3 may be integrated implicitly by the appraisal of relevance of the respective SLE, but were not measured directly. Disease-related alterations (level 5) were measured as long-term change in the distribution of leukocyte differentials. The definition of long-term change was based on the time-frame between baseline and follow-up assessment and consequential to the change in leukocyte differentials over the time frame of one year considered as temporal dynamics (level 7) over the time-frame of one year. Study 2 additionally aimed at assessing the HPA axis activation by the HCC (level 4) and long-term associations between the HCC and the leukocyte distribution considered as interactional dynamics (level 8).

4 Method

All data presented in this book were assessed as a part of the Dresden Burnout Study (DBS), a prospective cohort study which has been running in Dresden since January 2015. Data from two consecutive laboratory visits are provided, including the baseline assessment. The baseline assessment of biological markers (Bio_{T1}) was realized in Autumn/Winter 2015, the follow-up (Bio_{T2}) in Winter 2016/17.

Sampling: The study sample presented in this book is a subsample of the overall DBS study sample. The study pool includes all participants that registered via the study homepage (www.dresdner-burnout-studie.de) and is scattered Germany-wide. The study pool was recruited for the longitudinal online assessment of health-related questionnaire and demographic data with the aim of exploring risk factors and long-term consequences associated with burnout. It further aims at estimating the prevalence of burnout and/or work-related mental disorders (e.g. depression, anxiety disorder).

All the Dresden residents who registered via the DBS study homepage were invited to participate in the laboratory assessment of biomarkers in Dresden, which represents the recruitment procedure for the laboratory baseline sample (Bio_{T1}). The complete laboratory baseline sample (Bio_{T1}) was re-invited for a follow-up one year later (Bio_{T2}).

A detailed description of the design and methods of the DBS is provided by chapter 5 which outlines the study protocol for the first three-year study period, including the recruitment and assessment procedure of the study pool and the laboratory baseline sample. This book is based solely on data assessed during the laboratory sessions (subsample Bio_{T1} and Bio_{T2}).

Online data from the online study pool will be published elsewhere. The respective subsample characteristics, methods, and statistics are reported in detail in the method sections of Study 1 and Study 2.

5 The Dresden Burnout Study: Protocol of a prospective cohort study for the bio-psychological investigation of burnout

5.1 Introduction

According to the World Health Organization (WHO), work-related stress forms a growing health risk for western societies (Leka & Jain, 2010), pointing to the serious threat to both, the individual and the society. Up to twenty percent of the German population is affected by moderate to very high chronic stress. A variety of work-related parameters have been identified as main contributors to this high societal stress-level (Kocalevent, Klapp, Albani, & Brähler, 2013). A crucial condition in this context is burnout - a syndrome defined by (i) emotional and physical exhaustion, (ii) negative attitudes toward work, and a (iii) negative evaluation of one's work performance (Maslach et al., 2001; Shirom & Melamed, 2006). Studies on the epidemiology of burnout are scarce and restricted by the fact that burnout can be masked by other diagnoses like depression or chronic fatigue syndrome. Despite these conceptual challenges, there is a consensus that burnout is associated with immense economic costs, e.g., due to an increase in sick-leave (Bundespsychotherapeutenkammer, 2012; Korczak, Huber, & Kister, 2010). The burnout syndrome is considered a major risk factor for mental disorders (Ahola et al., 2005; Hakanen & Schaufeli, 2012) and physical diseases (Toker, Melamed, Berliner, Zeltser, & Shapira, 2012; Toppinen-Tanner, Ahola, Koskinen, & Väänänen, 2009), multiplying the burden for the individual and for the public health care system. Considering these consequences, surprisingly little is known about the etiology, course, and pathophysiology of burnout. Relatedly, research is hampered by the lack of an accepted syndrome definition or standardized diagnostic instruments (Korczak, Kister, & Huber, 2008). Only exhaustion is considered a sound psychological and physiological syndrome component (Kaschka, Korczak, & Broich, 2011). Given the above described situation, the Dresden Burnout Study (DBS) was initiated to advance the development of more effective screening methods which form the basis for future development of standardized prevention and treatment programs. Launched in January 2015, the DBS was designed as a prospective cohort study to assess burnout on a psychological, social, clinical, and biological level. The DBS is scheduled to run for 12 years with annually monitoring of up to 10.000 participants for psychometric and biological parameters. The present paper presents the study protocol and aims of the DBS and gives a brief overview of the first two assessment years.

5.1.1   Aims of DBS

The following paragraph will highlight the main aims of the DBS and give a brief overview of the current shortcomings of the burnout concept.

Aim 1: Understanding the development of symptoms and transition into burnout

So far, the burnout syndrome has primarily been described on the basis of cross-sectional studies, which does not allow for solid temporal and/or causal inferences about etiological factors of symptom development. The few available longitudinal studies show restricted generalizability of results by focusing on specific populations, e.g., middle-aged working women or employees of one single company (Evolahti, Hultell, & Collins, 2013; Leiter et al., 2013) or particular factors expected to cause burnout (Borritz et al., 2010; Lindwall, Gerber, Jonsdottir, Börjesson, & Ahlborg Jr, 2014). In addition, cross-sectional designs show a large symptom overlap of burnout with related disorders, primarily depression (Ahola et al., 2005; Bianchi, Boffy, Hingray, Truchot, & Laurent, 2013; Bianchi, Schonfeld, & Laurent, 2015; Hakanen & Schaufeli, 2012; Schonfeld & Bianchi, 2015). Based on these findings, burnout is widely believed not to be a syndrome by itself but rather a less stigmatizing label for depression. We hypothesize that symptom development within the burnout syndrome might be distinct from other disorders, even though cross-sectional symptomatology may show considerable overlap. In order to overcome the shortcomings of previous studies, longitudinal data from a larger sample are needed to understand a potential syndrome-specific progression of symptoms from work-stress to adverse health conditions.

Aim 2: Identifying biomarkers of burnout

Repeated assessments of potential burnout biomarkers may help to advance significantly the (differential) diagnosis of the syndrome and the individual trajectories of burnout from preclinical symptoms to clinical disease manifestation. According to a current meta-analysis (Danhof-Pont, van Veen, & Zitman, 2011; see also Grossi, Perski, Osika, & Savic, 2015), no reliable biomarker of burnout has been identified to date. This may be due to the rather small number of available studies and heterogenic study designs.

Due to its crucial role for the human stress response, the HPA axis and its regulation by GCs have been the main focus for systematic research on biomarkers in burnout so far (Mommersteeg, Heijnen, Verbraak, & van Doornen, 2006a, 2006b; Oosterholt, Maes, Van der Linden, Verbraak, & Kompier, 2015, 2016). By widespread central receptors, GCs can influence cognitive processes like learning and memory (Wolf, 2009) or exert effects on mood (Miller et al., 2007). Both aspects, cognition and mood regulation, seem to be pivotal for burnout development and progression (Grossi, et al., 2015; Maslach & Jackson, 1981). Furthermore, GCs have potent immuno-modulatory effects (Dhabhar, 2014; Hänsel et al., 2010; Rohleder, 2014), indicating a possible link between chronic stress in burnout and increased vulnerability to inflammatory or infectious diseases in burnout patients. Studies on burnout and immune parameters are scarce, but the available data consistently suggest reduced immune competence in affected individuals (Mommersteeg, Heijnen, Kavelaars, & van Doornen, 2006; von Känel et al., 2008).

Sex steroids have also been linked to burnout, although studies are scarce. Positive associations between burnout symptoms and testosterone levels were found in a study with a three-year follow-up (Grossi, Theorell, Jürisoo, & Setterlind, 1999). In contrast, a study by Grossi and colleagues from 2003 comparing two groups of women with high or low burnout symptomatology, respectively, revealed no differences between the groups for cortisol, progesterone, estradiol, or dehydroepiandrosterone-sulfate (Grossi et al., 2003). In accordance with these results, another study reported no associations between estradiol levels and burnout severity in either men or women (Lennartsson, Billig, & Jonsdottir, 2014).

Heart rate variability (HRV) is another valid starting point for the search of biological markers of burnout, given its frequently reported association with work-related stress (Jarczok et al., 2013). HRV is operationalized as the variability of time intervals between consecutive heart beats and is one of the most extensively studied indicators of autonomic nervous system (ANS) function (Task Force, 1996). The few existing studies on burnout, however, provide a contradictory picture with studies reporting either a reduction (de Vente, van Amsterdam, Olff, Kamphuis, & Emmelkamp, 2015), an elevation (Zanstra, Schellekens, Schaap, & Kooistra, 2006), or no differences in HRV (Jönsson et al., 2015) between individuals with burnout compared to controls.

Finally, the search for genes contributing to burnout vulnerability is warranted due to consistent reports of twin studies on the heritability of burnout symptoms (Mather, Bergström, Blom, & Svedberg, 2014; Middeldorp, Cath, & Boomsma, 2006). Using data from the Swedish twin cohort study including 20.286 individuals, Blom and colleagues (2012) concluded that genetic factors explain about one- third of the variance of individual differences in burnout symptoms. In addition, specific methylation patterns in candidate genes have been identified for burnout, linking epigenetic regulation with burnout vulnerability (Bakusic, Schaufeli, Claes, & Godderis, 2017). In consequence, genetic and epigenetic analyses are also incorporated into the biomarker assessment.

Taken together, the DBS aims to carefully evaluate a comprehensive set of promising biological markers for the risk, development and/or progression of burnout. Annual measurements over a total of 12 years will provide longitudinal data on the trajectories of biological markers in relation to burnout symptomatology. Different physiological systems such as the endocrine system, the immune system, the ANS as well as (epi)genetic markers will be examined (a detailed description of biomarkers is provided in section 5.3).

Aim 3: Paving the road for an improved definition of the burnout syndrome

Following aim 1, considering burnout as a specific diagnosis is currently still highly problematic. The classification systems DSM-5 (Diagnostic and Statistical Manual of Mental Disorders; American Psychiatric Association, 2013) and ICD-10 (International Classification of Disease; WHO, 1992) do not list burnout as a clinically relevant mental disorder. However, in the ICD-10, burnout is mentioned within the residual category Z 73 – *problems related to life management difficulty*. Importantly, burnout is listed within this residual category unrelated to symptoms or time criteria. For the definition of a burnout diagnosis meeting classification standards, a set of mandatory burnout symptoms and certain persistence criteria are needed. Such a diagnosis should demarcate burnout from other mental disorders such as depressive disorders or chronic fatigue syndrome (CFS; Bianchi et al., 2015; Huibers et al., 2003; Leone, Wessely, Huibers, Knottnerus, & Kant, 2011). Two examples for a standardized burnout diagnosis exist: The Swedish and the Dutch health systems provide standardized diagnoses that integrate burnout as a definable syndrome (Schaufeli, Leiter, & Maslach, 2009; Van Der Klink & Van Dijk, 2003). However, these approaches currently lack validation for an international transfer.

The DBS thus aims at identifying a burnout-specific set of symptoms. In addition, to identify a valid syndrome-specific time criterion, changes over time indicating remission, chronification, or relapse will be observed and linked to indicators of quality of life, impairment, and disability. Parallel to it, we will compare the results with those of standardized measurement instruments for depressive disorder and general fatigue to explore syndrome overlaps, transition, and comorbidities with burnout. Overall, this will allow for providing a criteria set for burnout, including differential diagnosis considerations.

Aim 4: Finding the commonalities between psychosocial factors associated with burnout

Over the last decades, several potentially burnout-associated psychosocial variables have been discussed with a particular focus on risk rather than protective factors. Predominantly, these either involve (work) environment factors or individual-level factors. With reference to the former, a recently published systematic review on psychosocial work conditions by Seidler and colleagues (2014) found quantitative job demands and increased job strain being most predictive for the emergence of burnout. On the individual level, personality and cognition are the most frequently studied concepts. With respect to personality, neuroticism and extraversion have most consistently been associated with burnout symptomatology (Alarcon, Eschleman, & Bowling, 2009; Swider & Zimmerman, 2010). The vast majority of studies on cognition revealed impairments to memory, executive function, and attention most consistently at severe stages of burnout symptomatology (Deligkaris, Panagopoulou, Montgomery, & Masoura, 2014).

In contrast to most of the previously conducted research, the DBS will simultaneously monitor different psychosocial variables on environmental and individual levels in a large, heterogeneous sample. With annual assessment waves, our aim is to identify those protective and risk factors with the strongest predictive value for burnout development and progression.

5.2   Materials and Methods

The study was approved by the local ethics committee and conducted in accordance with the Helsinki Declaration of 1975 as revised in 2008.

5.2.1 Sampling

The DBS is a prospective cohort study with a planned duration of 12 years. In annual examination waves psychological, social, and biological data will be collected. The primary aim of the first three years of the DBS is to build a large-scale sample (recruitment goal: 10.000 participants) within German-speaking countries, including an overlapping subsample that will be representative for the city of Dresden. To overcome a shortcoming of previous studies which focused predominately on very specific populations, inclusion criteria for the DBS are solely based on age (18-68) and adequate language skills (capable of reading and filling out questionnaires in German). Therefore, participants differing with respect to burnout symptomatology, professional and socioeconomic status as well as working area are recruited regardless of their individual work and stress antecedents. Subsequently, the sample will be stratified by demographics, burnout characteristics, and comorbidities (major depressive disorder, anxiety disorder, general fatigue). Medical conditions of participants are assessed but will not lead to exclusion. Burnout severity is measured with the Maslach Burnout Inventory-General Survey (MBI-GS; Büssing & Glaser, 1999; Schaufeli & Leiter, 1996), which is considered the gold standard for empirical burnout assessment.

5.2.2 Recruitment procedure

Two recruitment strategies are employed parallel to each other, as described below.

Sample 1: A convenient sample of participants who have been recruited by public media presence since January 2015. Participants´ recruitment is transmitted by heterogenic medial platforms. Furthermore, the DBS receives support from various companies and associations which inform associates and staff members about the DBS.

Sample 2: To decrease selection bias in our convenient sample, a second recruitment strategy was used for sample 2. Recruitment strategy for sample 1 implies a very heterogenic sample composition, which is the aim of the DBS. Indeed, it can be expected that people who already have a history of burnout, and/or are currently highly stressed, might respond to our medial recruitment rather than healthy people without any involvement with the study topic. To improve the generalizability of the study results, we included the supplementary sample 2. The recruitment phase for sample 2 was initiated from December 2016 to January 2017 via the population registry. The addresses of 10.000 private Dresden households were obtained from the Dresden City Registry by random sampling, and household members were informed about the DBS by postal invitation letters. In response to this effort, 850 participants (8.5%) have registered for study participation in the meantime. Even if we do not achieve a representative composition of Dresden residents with sample 2, the random drawing strategy will enlarge the generalizability of the results and will furthermore provide the first estimates of a burnout epidemiology in the city of Dresden.

5.2.3 *Registration and study homepage*

Study participation starts after registration to the DBS on our study homepage. The homepage further informs about participation formalities and provides information about help facilities and theoretical background about the burnout syndrome. The participants provide an e-mail address to which personalized log-in data are sent automatically. After the individual log-in and provision of their informed consent, the participants are recorded as DBS participants.

5.2.4 *Baseline and follow-up assessments*

The DBS subsumes online assessments of detailed questionnaire data and self-reported individual characteristics, lab-based sampling of biological markers as well as standardized clinical interview data. Figure 5 gives an overview of the cross-sectional and longitudinal DBS study design. A brief summary of the current sample characteristics is provided in Table 1.

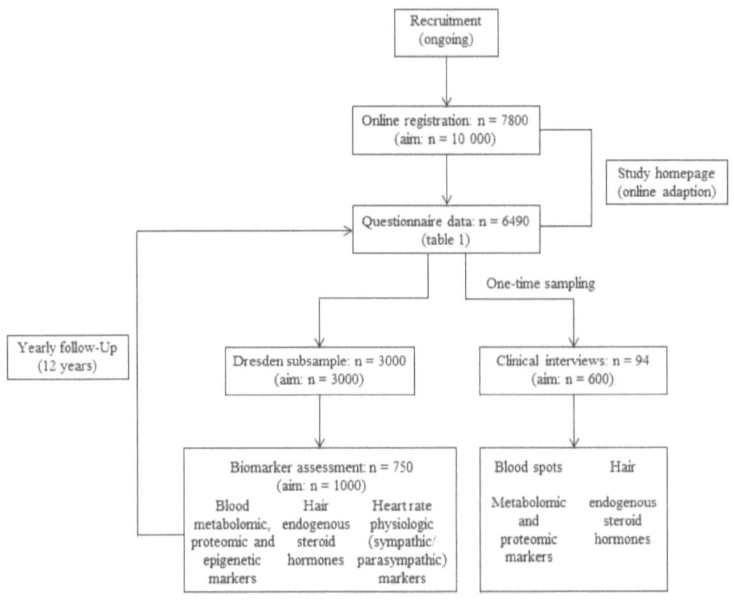

Figure 5. Flow chart of the prospective cohort study design of the Dresden Burnout Study.

After registration, the participants are invited to provide sociodemographic data and to complete a set of questionnaires (see Table 2) via the study homepage. After completion, automatized individual feedback is provided and can be downloaded from the homepage. The participants will be prompted to repeat the online questionnaire assessment, annually. We are aware that annual feedback about burnout and other health-related factors has to be considered a kind of intervention. The participants who complete the questionnaires yearly will receive regular feedback about their individual burnout and depression risk as well as about their sleep quality, behavioral work style, and health-related quality of life. Despite the consequence of a decrease in the generalizability of our results, we decided on this strategy for the benefit of a respectable sample size. Receiving individual feedback like regular risk assessment is expected to improve study involvement and compliance by working as a major

motivator for short- and long-term participation.

Table 1: Demoraphic and health-related characteristics of the DBS sample (N = 7058)

	M^a	Range
Age (years)	41.0 (11.5)	18-72
Sex (% female)	63.0	
BMI (kg/m²)	25.5 (5.1)	13.1-52.0
Underweight (%; BMI <18.5)	2.4	
Normal (%; BMI 18.5-24.9)	51.6	
Overweight (%; BMI 25-29.9)	29.0	
Obesity (%; BMI ≥30)	16.1	
Married/leaving with partner (%)	43.4	
Divorced (%)	5.7	
Currently employed (%)	89.0	
Main earner (%)	54.5	
Working hours per week	40.2 (10.9)	0.0-80.0
Additional side-job (%)	17.3	
Shift work (%)	14.0	
University degree (%)	52.4	
Income > 2000 € (net, %)	46.8	
Income < 1000 € (net, %)	16.4	
Current smokers (%)	23.1	
Duration smoking (years)	17.6	0.0-50.0
Constant medication (all, %)	45.1	
Burnout diagnose (lifetime, %)[b]	17.5	
MBI	2.4 (1.1)	0.0-6.0
PHQ-9	8.6 (5.5)	0.0-27.0
GAD-7	6.9 (4.9)	0.0-21.0

Note. Standard deviations are in parentheses. BMI = Body Mass Index; MBI = Maslach Burnout Inventory - General Survey total score; PHQ-9 = Patient Health Questionnaire sum score; GAD-7 = Generalized Anxiety Disorder 7
[a]Means and standard deviations in parentheses for metric measures; percentages for categorical measures.
[b]Phrasing: "Did a medical doctor or psychotherapist ever gave you the diagnosis of 'burnout'?"

For the purpose of an in-depth examination of burnout syndrome development and

associated comorbidities, we developed a burnout section for a standardized clinical interview

that was already tested successfully in a first pilot study with N = 94 participants (details will

be published elsewhere). The burnout section was added to the DIA-X/CIDI (Wittchen &

Pfister, 1997), which was modified for the DBS to be applied as computer-assisted telephone

interview (CATI). Since the CATI is going to be applied all over Germany, a stationary assessment of biological markers can only be assessed by biological samples which the participants were able to assess on their own and send to our institute (hair samples and dried blood spots). Albeit, after completing the clinical interview, the participants are asked to send hair samples for analysis (following guidelines for assessing hair samples provided to them; see below). Prospectively, dried blood spots will be included in the assessment of the interviewed subsample.

For the assessment of biological markers of burnout, the Dresden participants were invited for a first biomarker collection of hair samples, blood samples, and heart rate-measures in Autumn 2015 with a second study wave in Autumn 2016. Follow-ups will be repeated annually during a comparable time window to avoid seasonal effect confounding (Foster & Roenneberg, 2008).

5.2.4.1 Biomarker sampling procedure

All the Dresden participants (including sample 1 and sample 2) are invited via e-mail to participate in the laboratory session for biomarker assessment. The e-mail gives a brief process description, an estimate of the duration, and information about monetary compensation. After receiving the e-mail, the participants may choose the day and time for a study appointment on a calendar via the study homepage. The laboratory session includes reception and clarification, informed consent, biomarker sampling, and completion of a set of questionnaires (Table 2). The approximate duration of the procedure is 45 minutes. Figure 6 provides an overview of the procedure and the temporal sequence during the laboratory session.

5.2.5 *Self-report measures*

The DBS is the first prospective cohort study to assess burnout by using a variety of validated burnout questionnaires (see also Table 2). The MBI-GS (Schaufeli & Leiter, 1996)) was selected because of its importance to systematic burnout research. The 16 items are scored on three subscales (emotional exhaustion, cynicism, reduced personal efficacy). The response format for each item is a 7-point Likert scale with frequency ratings, ranging from 0 (never) to 6 (daily). Next, the *personal burnout* scale of the Copenhagen Burnout Inventory (CBI; Kristensen, Borritz, Villadsen, & Christensen, 2005) is added as further burnout estimate, which assesses burnout outside of a concrete work context. The CBI-scale comprises six items scoring on a 5-point Likert scale with frequency ratings from 1 (never/almost never) to 5 (always). As a third burnout measure, with reference to the Swedish burnout diagnosis (Beser et al., 2014), ICD-10 diagnostic criteria for *exhaustion disorder* (ED) are assessed as part of the DBS. More precisely, syndrome specificities are prompted employing four questions taken from Soderstrom, Jeding, Ekstedt, Perski, & Akerstedt, (2012).

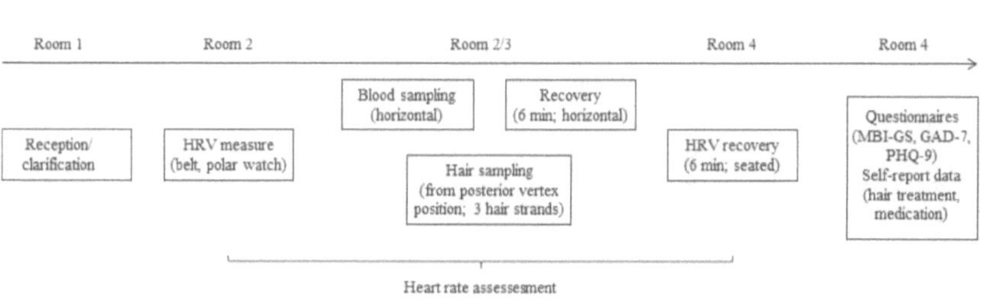

Figure 6. Flow chart of laboratory session for biomarker sampling of the Dresden Burnout Study.

Table 2: Questionnaire-based measures of the Dresden Burnout Study.

		Items	Scales
Burnout and related constructs			
Maslach Burnout Inventory-General Survey (Schaufeli & Leiter, 1996); German version (Büssing & Glaser, 1999)*	MBI-GS	16	Emotional exhaustion, cynicism, reduced personal efficacy
Copenhagen Burnout Inventory (Kristensen et al., 2005); German translation (Nübling et al., 2006)	CBI	6	Personal burnout
ICD-10 diagnosis for *exhaustion disorder* (Söderström et al., 2012)	ED	4	Exhaustion
Occupational Stress and Coping Inventory, short form (Schaarschmidt & Fischer, 1996)	AVEM	44	4 types of work-related coping-behaviors: type G (healthy ambitious), type S (unambitious), type A (tense), type B (exhausted/burned out)
Work environment factors			
Copenhagen Psychosocial Questionnaire (Kristensen et al., 2005), German version (Nübling et al., 2006)	COPSOQ	44	Emotional demands, work-privacy conflict, possibilities for development, role clarity, role conflict, social support, feedback at work, social relations, sense for community, harrassment, procedural justice, and job insecurity
Effort-reward imbalance questionnaire (Siegrist et al., 2004); short-form (Siegrist et al., 2009)	ERI	16	Effort, reward, over-commitment
Work-Home Interaction – Nijmegen (Geurts et al., 2005); German version (Nitzsche, 2011)	SWING	22	Negative work-home interaction, negative home-work interaction, positive work-home interaction, positive home-work interaction

Individual level factors

Big Five Inventory (John et al., 1991); German version; short form (Rammstedt & John, 2007)	BFI-10	10	Extraversion, agreeableness, conscientiousness, neuroticism, openness
General Self-Efficacy scale; German version (Schwarzer, 1993)	GSE	10	General self-efficacy
Locus of control; German short scale (Kovaleva et al., 2012)	IE-4	4	Internal and external locus of control
Perceived Stress Questionnaire (Levenstein et al., 1993); German short version (Fliege et al., 2001)	PSQ	20	Worries, tension, joy, demands
Need for Cognition; German scale (Bless et al., 1994)	NfC	16	Need for cognition

Health related factors and comorbidities

Patient Health Questionnaire, German version (Kroenke et al., 2001)*	PHQ-9	9	Depressive Disorder, screening
Generalized Anxiety Disorder Scale (Spitzer et al., 2006), German version (Löwe et al., 2008)*	GAD-7	7	General Anxiety Disorder, screening
SF-36 health survey (Ware et al., 2000), German translation (Bullinger et al., 1995)	SF-36	36	Physical functioning, role limitations because of physical health problems, bodily pain, social functioning, general mental health, role limitations because of emotional problems, vitality, general health perception
Pittsburg Sleep Quality Index, German translation (Backhaus et al., 2002)	PSQ-I	24	Subjective sleep quality, sleep latency, sleep duration, habitual sleep efficiency, sleep disturbances, use of sleep medication, daytime dysfunction

Finally, for the measurement of job-related experience and associated behavior outcomes, the 44-item short-form of the Occupational Stress and Coping Inventory (AVEM; Schaarschmidt & Fischer, 1996) is included. All items score on a 5-point rating scale (1 = completely disagree, 5 = completely agree). The AVEM sum score allows the allocation to one of four patterns of work-related copingbehaviors (type G = healthy ambitious, type S = unambitious, type A = tense, type B = exhausted/resigned) based on the maximal alignment with one's individual profile. Risk type A in its pure manifestation describes a person who "burns" for his/ her work, while the second risk type B can be considered as "burned out" at work (Schaarschmidt, 2006).

The decision to include a variety of burnout measures in the online assessment is rooted in the growing criticism about the current standard of assessing burnout solely on basis of the Maslach Burnout Inventory. Critical aspects are, e.g., the lack of clinical validity (Kleijweg, Verbraak, & Van Dijk, 2013), a tautological syndrome definition (Kristensen et al., 2005), and a considerable overlap with other syndromes, or general exhaustion (Maslach & Leiter, 2016a). By a simultaneous assessment of alternative burnout measures, our aim is to extract key factors that describe the burnout syndrome on the continuum between mild and clinical burnout and demarcate it from related diseases. For an assessment of comorbidities and/or overlaps, screening questionnaires for related diseases are included as well as general health measures. Furthermore, instruments assessing the work environment and individual trait and state factors are also included, based on validity and comparability considerations.

5.2.6 *Assessment of biological burnout markers*

5.2.6.1 Endocrine biomarkers

The DBS involves annual assessments of different steroid hormones, e.g., cortisol, cortisone, testosterone, progesterone, dehydroepiandrosterone, and estradiol, from hair and blood serum specimens. Hair steroid analyses comprise a recently developed method that allows capturing stress-related changes in long-term patterns of hormone secretion (Stalder et al., 2017). For hormone extraction from hair, strains are cut scalp-near at the posterior vertex position. Hormones are determined from the 3 cm- segment most proximal to the scalp as an index of cumulative output over the preceding three-month period (Stalder et al., 2012) and quantified using the gold-standard liquid-chromatography tandem mass spectrometry approach (Gao, Kirschbaum, Grass, & Stalder, 2016; Gao et al., 2013).

5.2.6.2   Immunologic biomarkers

The HPA axis regulates the availability of GCs, which in turn interact with immune parameters. As a consequence, due to the stress reactiveness of the HPA axis, immune functions can be influenced by chronic stress conditions (Dhabhar, 2014; Dhabhar & Mcewen, 1997; Glaser & Kiecolt-Glaser, 2005). This also indicates that immune parameters are likely to be sensitive to the conditions of burnout (Hänsel et al., 2010). In the DBS, the immune parameters are annually collected via EDTA blood tubes. With the longitudinal assessment of the immune parameters, we aim at further exploring the link between burnout and disease processes, including the potential shift from immune competence to immune suppression (Dhabhar, 2014) that may accompany this condition.

5.2.6.3   Physiologic biomarkers

Given that the ANS is known to primarily be involved in the regulation of stress reactivity, astonishingly little research has been carried out investigating burnout-associated alterations in the autonomic function. HRV, defined as beat-to-beat variations in the timing of heart beats, is used in the DBS to examine the role of the ANS in burnout diseases. More precisely, inter-beat intervals are recorded with a Polar RS800 CX system via the corresponding chest belt (Polar Electro OY, Kempele, Finland) from all participants during biomarker sampling procedures. The data are transferred to the Polar Precision Performance

Software (Polar Electro OY, Kempele, Finland) and subsequently artefact-corrected according to the guidelines of the Task Force of the European Society of Cardiology and the North American Society of Pacing and Electrophysiology (1996).

On the grounds of previous findings that certain dysregulations in biological systems become evident only under specific experimental conditions (Kudielka & Wüst, 2010), HRV is analyzed during different measurement occasions, namely an emotionally-arousing situation (blood sampling), a recumbent recovery period directly after blood sampling, and a resting condition while seated (6 minutes each).

5.2.6.4   Genetic and epigenetic biomarkers

Several relevant candidate genetic variations for burnout have been identified by genome-wide association studies such as in the melatonin receptor 1A gene or in the intron of uronyl-2-sulfotransferase (rs13219957; Sulkava et al., 2013, 2017). These results provide promising avenues for better identifying people with an increased susceptibility to burnout and corresponding allocations to prevention programs. Furthermore, epigenetic analyses will be conducted focusing on the glucocorticoid receptor gene (NR3C1) and brain-derived neurotrophic factor (BDNF) which have been reported to display different methylation patterns in chronic stress and depression, while the serotonin transporter gene (SLC6A4) methylation was similarly affected by chronic stress, burnout, and depression (Bakusic et al., 2017). Therefore, the longitudinal prospective assessment of changes in the methylation patterns of key genes in large samples is needed to clarify the role of epigenetic regulation in burnout.

5.2.7   *Why focusing on the assessment of biomarkers of burnout?*

Even if previous studies suggest physiological alterations to be involved in burnout, a ground base for specific biomarkers is still missing. Most results are single findings and lack comparability and replication. The majority of biomarker-based burnout studies assessed endocrine alterations mainly on the level of the HPA axis but with huge variability in study protocols. Summarizing, up to date, there is no biomarker that can be considered a prime candidate in burnout research (Danhof-Pont et al., 2011). On the other hand, there is sound evidence that burnout enters the body somehow and acts as a risk factor for physical illness, e.g., cardiovascular disease (Toker et al., 2012), Type 2 diabetes (Melamed et al., 2006), vascular dementia (Andel et al., 2012), and a shortened life cycle (Ahola et al., 2010). Furthermore, decades of stress research provide a solid ground for potential pathways of stress/body interactions (e.g. Dhabhar, 2014; Glaser & Kiecolt-Glaser, 2005; Kudielka, Schommer, Hellhammer, & Kirschbaum, 2004; Miller et al., 2007; Rohleder, 2012), and even though a standardized definition and diagnosis for the burnout syndrome is still missing (Kaschka et al., 2011), there is no doubt that burnout sufferers experience a significant level of stress. A major challenge in the search for burnout biomarkers is the anticipated overlap with other syndromes. Together with a close self-report assessment it is our aim to find patterns of psychological and biological data which are specific to burnout and distinguishable from other syndromes (e.g. depression), or general exhaustion (Maslach & Leiter, 2016a). In line with Maslach and Leiter (2016b) we expect that burnout is not merely an equivalent of exhaustion and aim at evaluating potential burnout patterns with specific biological outcomes.

5.3   Results

The DBS started in January 2015. Since then, data are consecutively generated. An initial cross-sectional analysis of the DBS data supports the idea of burnout-associated autonomic dysfunction, indicated by reduced vagally-mediated HRV in individuals with an elevated burnout symptomatology (Kanthak et al., 2017). An upcoming analysis of longitudinal data will give further insight into the replicability and questions of causality regarding the observed effect. Recently published data on associations between the HCC and the burnout symptomatology by Penz, Stalder, et al. (2018) suggest alterations on the level of the HPA axis. Burnout measured with a dichotomous classifier (high versus no/medial burnout symptomatology) was positively related to the HCC, indicating hypercortisolism in individuals who suffer from chronic stress in burnout.

As the DBS is still in its initial stage, no longitudinal data is currently available. First cross-sectional analyses focused solely on potential burnout biomarkers, as the DBS declares its emphasis on the research of physiological consequences of burnout or work-related stress. Indeed, within the following months, baseline and follow-up questionnaire data will be available and will provide first insight into risk and health factors, overlaps, patterns, and comorbidities. Longitudinal biomarker and online-questionnaire data will provide a sound basis for understanding the burnout syndrome with its specific antecedents and consequences. The collected data will help to clarify if burnout is a syndrome on its own with a syndrome-specific symptomatology and specific treatment requirements or rather a new word for already well -established diseases (e.g. depression or CFS).

5.4   Discussion

The DBS aims at closing the empirical gap between myth, unstandardized, intuitive clinical practice, and personal opinions about the burnout syndrome, on the one hand, and the detrimental consequences that this condition is likely to have for a number of individuals, on the other hand. The aim is a longitudinal assessment of a potential burnout development on the symptom and syndrome level, with a synchronous monitoring of biological markers which might precede, co-occur, or follow burnout development. Annual assessment waves over a total of 12 years will provide a unique opportunity for investigating burnout symptom trajectories in relation to underlying neurobiological changes. This should further provide a sound basis for preventive policies and treatment of the burnout syndrome. Ensuing advancements in the prediction of burnout risk and course will further enable a more accurate handling and resource allocation in the early stages of this condition. For example, the identification of potential biological markers of burnout might complement screening options for burnout susceptibility and help to validate the diagnosis. Thus, given the large sample size and the prospective-longitudinal study design, this study might pave the road for a comprehensive characterization of burnout and a potential for an internationally accepted burnout diagnosis.

6 *Study I:* Hair cortisol concentrations as a biological marker for burnout symptomatology

6.1 <u>Introduction</u>

Work-related chronic stress is a major health challenge in Western societies, often leading to burnout as a hallmark consequence. Burnout is defined by increased levels of emotional exhaustion (EE), reduced efficacy (rE), and cynical attitudes (Cy) towards work (Maslach et al., 2001). Besides these psychological responses to chronic work overload, individuals suffering from burnout often show comorbidity with type II diabetes, disorder of lipid metabolism, allergies as well as cardiovascular and musculoskeletal problems (Melamed, Shirom, Toker, Berliner, & Shapira, 2006; Toppinen-Tanner et al., 2009). One potential mechanism linking burnout to these adverse health conditions is an altered activity of the HPA axis, with changes in the GC output as a consequence of chronic stress. Despite a myriad of studies on stress and cortisol published in the past decades, surprisingly few studies sofar have examined alterations of GC levels in relation to burnout. These published data are rather inconsistent with reports of both, hyper- and hypo-cortisolism (reviewed in Danhof-Pont et al., 2011). The heterogeneous findings might in part be due to methodological limitations of these studies, as mainly spot measurements were employed, using only a few or even one single blood or saliva sample. These specimens are particularly sensitive to transient fluctuations in the HPA axis activity (Spiga et al., 2014) and may, thus, not reflect the GC output over prolonged periods of time. In contrast, GC assessment in human scalp hair extracts provides an integrative measure of cortisol, which allows a retrospective analysis of the HPA activity over several months prior to hair collection. Accordingly, there is strong evidence to suggest that hair cortisol (hairF) concentration is a valid and solid index of long-term glucocorticoid secretion, with high intraindividual stability and test-retest reliability (Stalder et al., 2017). In the present study, we thus employed hairF as a potential biomarker for burnout symptoms. In addition, concentrations of cortisone in hair (hairE) were measured simultaneously to obtain a more robust GC index (Stalder et al., 2013), and the sum of hairE and hairF (hairEF$_{sum}$) was implemented as a further GC estimate. Burnout was assessed by a global burnout score as well as by subscales representing the three dimensions of burnout (EE, Cy, rE) *sensu* Maslach et al. (2001). To control for potential confounding effects of a burnout/ depressivity overlap, a screening scale for depressive symptomatology was also administered.

6.2   <u>Materials and methods</u>

6.2.1   Participants

The participants were a subsample of the DBS, a large-scale cohort study with annual study waves for biomarker sampling that was approved by the local ethics committee and conducted in accordance with the Declaration of Helsinki. The DBS participants had been recruited through different public media platforms in Germany with an emphasis on the Dresden region. Inclusion criteria were being aged between 18 and 68, sufficient language skills to fill out German questionnaires, and no current pregnancy. The presented data are based on the results of the first wave of biomarker sampling that was conducted from September to October 2015. All the participants living in Dresden were invited to participate. Out of 1.864 invited participants, 446 accepted our invitation, which resulted in N = 344 hair samples for analysis (due to insufficient hair lengths or refusal to contribute a hair strand). Due to quantification limits of the assay method (at least 0.1 pg/mg per sample), the final dataset was comprised of 314 participants (mean ± SD age: 41.65 ± 11.26; 16.2% male). The participants were compensated with a gift voucher worth 15 euros.

6.2.2   Procedure

The participants completed the questionnaires through the study homepage one week prior to sampling. By using a personalized log-in, each participant completed information about sociodemographic and health-related factors as well as on burnout and depressive symptomatology before attending the laboratory session. Biomarker sampling took place between 8 am and 7 pm with an average duration of 50 minutes. Besides hair collection, the lab sessions included an assessment of the HRV and a blood draw (data not reported here).

6.2.3   Glucocorticoid analysis

The hair strands were cut as close as possible to the scalp from a posterior vertex position. HairF and hairE concentrations were determined from the 3 cm-segment most proximal to the scalp. Given an average hair growth of 1 cm per month (Wennig, 2000), this segment represents the cumulated GC secretion over a 3-month period prior to sampling. The washing procedure and GC extraction followed the laboratory protocol described by Gao et al. (2013). All the samples were analyzed by liquid chromatography coupled with tandem mass spectrometry (LC-MS/MS).

6.2.4   Self-report measures

Information about hair-specific characteristics and treatment (shampooing per week, natural hair color, curls, permanent wave, and coloration) as well as about sociodemographic, anthropometric, and health-related variables (sex, age, body mass index, smoking status, alcohol and caffeine intake, medication intake) were assessed through a self-developed questionnaire. Burnout symptoms were assessed with the German Version of the MBI-GS (Büssing & Glaser, 1999). The MBI-GS consists of 16 items that can be subsumed to one general burnout factor (MBI total score) or separate scores for three scales (emotional exhaustion: EE, cynicism: Cy, reduced efficacy: rE), respectively. Internal consistency was considered adequate for all subscales (EE: $\alpha = 0.92$; Cy: $\alpha = 0.85$; rE: $\alpha = 0.85$), and for the average of the 16 items (MBI total: $\alpha = 0.90$; all 446 participants included in the analyses). A dichotomous classification of burned-out participants (MBI_{dicho}) was performed by dividing the MBI total score into "severe burnout symptoms" (MBI total score ≥ 3.5) versus "no or moderate symptoms" (MBI total score < 3.5; Kalimo, Pahkin, Mutanen, & Toppinen-Tanner, 2003). To obtain information on depressivity, we used the Patient Health Questionnaire (PHQ-9) German Version (Löwe, Spitzer, Zipfel, & Herzog, 2002), a 9-item screening instrument for major depression. Furthermore, a dichotomous classification of potentially depressed participants (PHQ_{dicho}) was computed by dividing the PHQ-9 total score into "moderate to severe major depression" (total score > 14) versus "no or mild major depression" (total score ≤ 14; Kroenke, Spitzer, & Williams, 2001).

6.2.5 Data pre-processing and statistical analyses

HairF, hairE, and $hairEF_{sum}$ were log-transformed to approach a normal distribution. Extreme log-transformed values (± 3 standard deviations from the mean) were excluded, leaving a total of n = 305 hair samples for the analyses. Associations between questionnaire scores and GC measures were examined by simple regression analyses. To control for potential confounders, sequential multiple regression analyses were conducted to examine the predictive value of each burnout and depressivity variable towards hairF, hairE, and $hairEF_{sum}$, respectively. As a first step, potential confounders were entered *en bloc* into the model: sex, age, BMI, hair treatment, alcohol consumption, smoking, caffeine consumption and medication intake (Stalder et al., 2017). As a second step the burnout score was added to the baseline model. Considering the collinearity of the MBI total score variables and the three MBI subscales (all rs between 0.40 and 0.89), separate analyses were conducted for the MBI total score, each MBI subscale (EE, Cy, and rE), and for the classifier MBI_{dicho}. As burnout and depressivity are characterized by overlapping symptomatology, we conducted subsequent sensitivity analyses to explore the predictive value of depression variables for hairF, hairE, and hairEF$_{sum}$. This was carried out by using the same baseline model, but added both, the depressivity and the burnout predictors in a second and a third step, respectively. Finally, potential mediating effects of sex were investigated separately for simple regression analyses. Significance was defined by a threshold of $\alpha = 0.05$ (two-sided). All the analyses were conducted using IBM SPSS Statistics 22 (SPSS Inc., IL, USA).

Table 3: Demographic and clinical sample characteristics.

	M (SD)	Range
Demographics		
Age, year	41.76 (11.31)	20 - 64
Female (%)	235 (83.90)	
Body mass index (kg/m²)	24.69 (4.30)	17.30 – 41.77
Hair-related variables		
Washes per week	3.52 (1.86)	1 - 7
Curls (%)	122 (43.60)	
Coloration (%)	112 (40.00)	
Permanent wave (%)	9 (3.30)	
Clinical characteristics		
MBI total score	2.24 (1.16)	0.12 – 4.73
MBI$_{dicho}$;"high burnout" (%)	50 (17.90)	
Emotional exhaustion (EE)	2.87 (1.59)	0 - 6
Cynicism (Cy)	2.02 (1.55)	0 - 6
Reduced efficacy (rE)	4.38 (1.15)	0 - 23
PHQ-9	8.37 (5.14)	0 - 23
PHQ$_{dicho}$ "serious MD" (%)	37 (13.20)	

Note. standard errors are in parentheses. MBI total score = Maslach Burnout Inventory – General Survey; EE, Cy, and rE = MBI sub score; MBI$_{dicho}$ = dichotomized MBI score; PHQ-9 = Patient Health Questionnaire sum score; PHQ$_{dicho}$ = dichotomized PHQ-9 score

6.3 Results

Table 3 shows the demographic, hair-related, and clinical characteristics of the sample. The results of the regression analyses showing the predictive value of burnout measures (MBI total score, EE, Cy, rE, MBI$_{dicho}$) and depression scores (PHQ-9 sum score, PHQ$_{dicho}$) on hairF, hairE and hairEF$_{sum}$ are provided in Table 4. Among the burnout scores, the classifier MBI$_{dicho}$ predicted all the GC measures (hairF: $R^2 = 0.02$, $F_{(1,279)} = 6.22$, $p = 0.01$; hairE: $R^2 =$

0.02, $F_{(1,300)}$ = 6.13, p = 0.01; hairEF$_{sum}$: R^2 = 0.02, $F_{(1,289)}$ = 5.08, p = 0.03). The results remained significant for hairF and hairE after fully controlling for potential confounders (hairF: β = 0.14, t = 2.20, p = 0.03; hairE: β = 0.13, t = 2.15, p = 0.03), and as a trend for hairEF$_{sum}$ (β = 0.11, t = 1.81, p = 0.07). The rE subscale predicted hairF (R^2 = 0.02, $F_{(1,279)}$ = 6.06, p = 0.01) in the simple regression as well as hairEF$_{sum}$ in the simple (R^2 = 0.03, $F_{(1,289)}$ = 7.90, p < 0.01) and multiple (β = -0.13, t = 2.03, p = 0.04) regression. However, no such association with hairE was detected. No significant associations emerged with overall burnout symptoms (MBI total score) or the MBI subscale EE and Cy. Similarly, none of the depressivity measures explained the variance in hairF, hairE or hairEF$_{sum}$.

Table 4: Summary of regression coefficients.

	hairF		hairE		hairEF$_{sum}$	
	simple regression	multiple regression	simple regression	multiple regression	simple regression	multiple regression
MBI	.10 (.02)	.09 (.02)	.06 (.02)	.04 (.02)	.10 (.02)	.08 (.02)
EE	.03 (.02)	.02 (.02)	<.01 (.01)	<.01 (.01)	.02 (.01)	<.01 (.01)
Cy	.11 (.02)	.11 (.02)	.09 (.01)	.09 (.01)	.10 (.01)	.10 (.01)
rE	.15 (.02)*	.12 (.02)°	.09 (.02)	.04 (.02)	.16 (.02)**	.13 (.02)*
MBI$_{dicho}$	.15 (.06)*	.14 (.07)*	.14 (.05)*	.13 (.05)*	.13 (.05)*	.11 (.06)°
PHQ-9	.07 (.01)	.04 (.01)	-.01 (< .01)	-.05 (<.01)	.05 (<.01)	<.01 (<.01)
PHQ$_{dicho}$	.08 (.07)	.02 (.08)	-.02 (.05)	-.07 (.06)	.07 (.06)	<.01 (.06)

Note. Standard errors are in parentheses. MBI = Maslach Burnout Inventory – General Survery total score, EE = emotional exhaustion, Cy = cynicism, rE = reduced efficacy, MBI$_{dicho}$ = dichotomous burnout variable, PHQ-9 = screening for major depression, PHQ$_{dicho}$ = dichotomous depression variable. N = 305, [1]pg/mg, logarithmized
*p < .05; **p < .01; °trend ($p \leq$ .07)

All the reported significances for the predictive value of MBI$_{dicho}$ remained significant after fully adjusting for PHQ (MBI$_{dicho}$/hairF: ΔR^2 = 0.02 for step 3, p = 0.03; MBI$_{dicho}$/hairE: ΔR^2 = 0.03, p < 0.01; MBI$_{dicho}$/hairEF$_{sum}$: ΔR^2 = 0.02, p = 0.05) and PHQ$_{dicho}$ (MBI$_{dicho}$/hairF: ΔR^2 = 0.02, p = 0.02; MBI$_{dicho}$/hairE: ΔR^2 = 0.03, p < 0.01; MBI$_{dicho}$/hairEF$_{sum}$: ΔR^2 = 0.02, p = 0.05). Sex was no significant moderator of the GC-burnout associations which were detected using simple regression analyses (hairF/rE*sex: R^2 = 0.02, ΔR^2 < 0.01, p = 0.41; hairEFsum/rE*sex: R^2 = 0.03, ΔR^2 < 0.01, p = 0.34; hairF/MBI$_{dicho}$*sex: R^2 = 0.03, ΔR^2 =

0.01, $p = 0.12$; hairE/MBI$_{dicho}$*sex: $R^2 = 0.03$, $\Delta R^2 = 0.01$, $p = 0.10$; hairFE$_{sum}$/MBI$_{dicho}$*sex: $R^2 = 0.03$, $\Delta R^2 = 0.01$, $p = 0.09$).

6.4 <u>Discussion</u>

This is the first study to report associations between hairF and hairE concentrations and burnout. We found hypercortisolism in individuals who reported a significant number of burnout symptoms. Associations became stronger when burnout was measured with the classifier MBI$_{dicho}$. Our results are consistent with previous meta-analytic studies that suggest an increase in the basal GC secretion under chronic stress (Miller et al., 2007, Stalder et al., 2017).

Interestingly, comparable associations did not appear when burnout was measured with the continuous MBI total score. At first glance, it seems surprising that MBI$_{dicho}$ significantly contributes to hairF and hairE, while the continuous MBI total score does not. Due to the loss of individual information and the consequential reduction of power, dichotomization can hardly 'improve' the prediction of an outcome (MacCallum, Zhang, Preacher, & Rucker, 2002) whenever the functional form of the statistical model is correctly specified. We therefore hypothesize that the association between burnout and GC exposure is more appropriately described by a nonlinear relationship: burnout symptoms may not affect basal GC levels until a certain level of severity is transcended, whereas burnout symptoms in the upper severity range would hardly unfold any additional impact on the GCs. Nonlinear relationships between burnout symptoms and GC alterations might also provide a framework for explaining contrary results reporting decreased salivary cortisol in burned-out individuals (e.g. Juster et al., 2011; Marchand, Juster, Durand, & Lupien, 2014). It can be speculated, that GC alterations develop as a function of time with a potential change from hyper- to hypocortisolism or vice versa. Accordingly, prospective data will become mandatory for understanding the time-course of biological alterations in burnout (Juster et al., 2011).

Consequently, considering the immune modulating effect of the GC (Dhabhar, 2014), the link between burnout and immune deficits (as shown e.g. for allergies or type II diabetes) via GC alterations needs to be examined in further studies. Future studies should compile detailed intra-individual information about the severity and duration associated with burnout symptoms. Based on that information, it should be tested if there is a change point, where symptom severity and duration start to significantly alter basal GC secretion and further immune competence.

Surprisingly, the association between burnout and hairF or hairE were hardly attributable to subscale *emotional exhaustion* (EE), although Maslach and colleagues (2001) considered EE the core dimension of burnout. By contrast, *reduced efficacy* (rE) was significantly associated with increased hairF and hairE values. It remains to be found out if rE represents a consequence of EE at a later syndrome stage, where individuals are already more vulnerable to GC alterations. Moreover, it remains to be determined if potential change points exist for EE, Cy, and rE, thereby providing a valid basis for applying cut-off values for MBI subscales.

Given the close link between burnout symptoms and depression (reviewed in Bianchi et al., 2015), we included a self-report screening measure for major depression (MD). Inconsistent with previous research on spot GC measurement (Miller et al., 2007), but consistent with findings in hair cortisol (Stalder et al., 2017), we found no specific associations between the MD symptoms and hairF or hairE. This further supports the notion that emotional exhaustion – the burnout symptom most closely linked to depression – is unlikely to be the main driver of the reported associations. Nonetheless, it is an interesting prospect for future studies to provide detailed clinical life-time information about the severity and course of depressive symptoms. The same is advisable for burnout symptoms. Both syndromes should further be compared by their life-time symptomatology and interactional impact on psychological and biological level. In conclusion, the findings of the present study provide first tentative evidence for hairF and hairE alterations in burnout. Based on our results, we hypothesize a potential change point, where general symptom severity starts to interfere with basal GC levels.

7 *Study II:* Stressful life events predict one-year change of leukocyte composition in peripheral blood

7.1 <u>Introduction</u>

More than 65% of all individuals worldwide experience at least one traumatic event during their life-time (Benjet et al., 2016). Trauma experience can be based on stressful life events (SLE) like an unexpected death of a loved one, criminal offenses including robbery and rape, experience of life-threatening illnesses, or traffic accidents (Benjet et al., 2016). SLE can happen to everybody at any time, and it seems plausible that these experiences may affect an individual long after stress cessation. Exposure to a SLE furthermore increases the risk for subsequent adverse life experiences (Benjet et al., 2016), for example, as caused by secondary stressors (e.g. poverty as a consequence of property loss due to a natural disaster; Lock et al., 2012). It has been shown that experiencing a stressful life event augments the risk for adverse mental health consequences (Beards et al., 2013; Cattaneo et al. 2015; Danese et al., 2008; Kendler, Karkowski, & Prescott, 1999; Kraan, Velthorst, Smit, de Haan, & van der Gaag, 2015; Tennant, 2002). Besides the challenge of an individual's mental health, exposure to SLE might also contribute to the variation in physical health (Glaser & Kiecolt-Glaser, 2005). Even if the underlying pathways of a link between SLE and health/disease are not fully understood, epidemiological research consistently suggests associations between SLE and negative health outcomes, e.g., arthritis (Keyes et al., 2013), heart disease, diabetes (Scott et al., 2013), and inflammatory disorders like asthma and atopic dermatitis (Kilpeläinen et al., 2002). Oilman and Siegel (1996) demonstrated in a sample of 3,132 adults that the risk for chronic physical malfunctioning increased 3-fold if the person reported at least one life-time stressful event. Likewise, SLE have been discussed as one major factor that accounts for inequalities in the human population according to disease, illness, and mortality, comparable with the socioeconomic status (Pearlin, Schieman, Fazio, & Meersman, 2005). The relevance of SLE for adverse mental and physical health outcomes is further underlined by the observation of a cumulative increase of disease with the number of SLE a person experienced (Scott et al., 2013; Turner & Lloyd, 1995). Thus, there is suggestive evidence that (cumulative) life stress can leave physical 'scars' that render an individual more vulnerable to a variety of adverse health conditions over the life-span.

7.2 Psychophysiological background

The immunosuppression theory represents one theoretical framework to explain the above outlined associations between SLE and adverse health outcomes. The underlying assumption is that sustained stress heightens the risk for adverse health outcomes by suppressing the immune response, leaving the host vulnerable for disease pathogenesis (Miller, Cohen, & Ritchey, 2002). A potential pathway for immuno-suppression as a consequence of SLE can be explained by the GCR model (Cohen et al., 2012; Cole, 2008; Miller et al., 2002; Miller, Rohleder, Stetler, & Kirschbaum, 2005). The GCR model is based on the premise that chronic stress diminishes the immune systems sensitivity to GC hormones that normally terminate the inflammatory cascade. An initial exposure to high GC levels leads to a counter-regulatory mechanism at level of white blood cells (WBCs), that downregulate the expression and/or function of GC-binding receptors. As a consequence, GCs lose their place of activity and CG-regulated dampening of inflammation might be impaired (Miller et al., 2002). Evidence for the GCR model is provided by many animal and human studies, underpinning that the HPA axis and, thus, the availability of the GC cortisol can be influenced by negative events and emotions (review: Miller et al., 2007). Likewise, life stress probably contributes to the peripheral distribution of WBCs, resulting for instance in a decline in lymphocyte proliferation (review: Segerstrom & Miller, 2004). Several authors have speculated that GC and immune alterations due to stress exposure outlast the event and become irreversible at a certain level of stress severity and duration, for example, by linking adverse childhood experiences to health consequences in later life (reviews: Baumeister, Akhtar, Ciufolini, Pariante, & Mondelli, 2015; Coelho, Viola, Walss-Bass, Brietzke, & Grassi-Oliveira, 2014). The SLE are indicative of psychological distress which generally is neither transient nor persistent in a classical sense. Exposure to SLE can affect a person's life in a way that goes far beyond the event, e.g., by rumination about the negative event (Garnefski, Kraaij, & Spinhoven, 2001) or grief and reorganization of live and self (Gillies & Neimeyer, 2006). Therefore, individuals who experienced an SLE might suffer from a steady, chronic stress load following the event even after stress cessation.

7.2.1   *HPA axis alterations and immune defence*

The HPA axis and the immune system are bi-directionally interwoven, representing two constantly interacting systems. GC receptors are expressed on most immune cells (Cain & Cidlowski, 2017), and GCs have the potential to suppress inflammation by switching off multiple inflammatory genes that code for cytokines, chemokines, adhesion molecules, inflammatory enzymes, or receptors (Barnes & Adcock, 2009). They modulate immuno-enhancing as well as immuno-suppressive effects (Cain & Cidlowski, 2017; Franchimont, et al., 2002; Sapolsky et al., 2000) at the level of the innate/adaptive immune response (Franchimont et al., 2002). Furthermore, monokines and cytokines, including IL-1, IL-6, or TNF, stimulate the hypothalamus leading to HPA axis activation and an increased availability of cortisol (Cain & Cidlowski, 2017).

GCs can curb leukocyte migration by the production of several chemokines and chemo-attractants and by direct GC receptor binding to chemokine-encoding mRNA transcripts. They can further influence the peripheral blood flow and leukocyte cell death (Cain & Cidlowski, 2017), which might affect the total number of circulating WBCs. The susceptibility of WBCs to GCs was shown by Dhabhar and colleagues (2012) via exposing rodents to a 120 min restraint stressor. Neutrophils, for example, showed a 45% increase during the first 6 min of stress exposure and a 75% increase after 120 min stress exposure. Contrarily, lymphocytes reached a peak of 26% increase after 6 min stress, following by a subsequent decline. After 120 min of restrained stress, lymphocytes showed a 45% decrease. Monocytes did not alter significantly during stress exposure. Hormone injection with GCs resulted in a significant decrease of monocyte and lymphocyte numbers that was not observed in neutrophils. Further rodent data on cumulative stress were reported by Engler and colleagues (2004). They showed that repeated social defeat (using the social disruption, SDR, paradigm; Avitsur, Stark, & Sheridan, 2001) altered the neutrophil and monocyte distribution in the bone marrow, peripheral blood, and spleen of male mice. The increase in the total number of circulating neutrophils and monocytes in peripheral blood became more pronounced, the more SDR cycles a mouse was exposed to. After six cycles over six consecutive days, circulating neutrophil numbers increased 5-fold compared with controls, monocytes by a factor of two, suggesting that cumulative stress exposure enlarges the stress-regulated immune adaption.

The total number of WBCs and their subsets (neutrophils, lymphocytes, monocytes) from peripheral blood, represent a basic parameter for detecting the activation of the immune system and inflammation (Vozarova et al., 2002). Even if normal ranges are quite large, a correct proportion of immune cell types can indicate a proper immune defense (Segerstrom & Miller, 2004). Maladaptive WBC alterations are associated with several adverse health conditions like diabetes (Vozarova et al., 2002), stroke (Christensen & Boysen, 2004), and death after a myocardial infarction (Horne et al., 2005). It may be speculated that GC-driven alterations in the peripheral distribution of the WBCs are at the basis of an increased vulnerability to disease.

7.2.2 Research agenda

In line with the above explained GCR model we hypothesize that the cumulative SLE a person faces during his or her life promotes a maladaptive immune defense which might further lead to a higher vulnerability to several adverse inflammatory and health conditions. We expect GC-mediated alterations in the WBCs to be one major source for higher disease vulnerability in individuals affected by SLE.

Based on a large cohort study of stressed individuals, we examined WBCs (neutrophils, lymphocytes, and monocytes) at first visit (T1) and 1-year follow-up (T2) in association with cumulative SLE experience. GCs were measured as hair cortisol concentrations (HCC) at both time points, which serve as a marker for cumulative 3-month cortisol secretion. Considering that inflammation has reciprocal effects on lymphopoiesis and granulopoiesis in the bone morrow (Ueda et al., 2005; Ueda et al., 2004), we additionally considered the neutrophil/lymphocyte ratio in our analyses. Our research model is summarized in Figure 7.

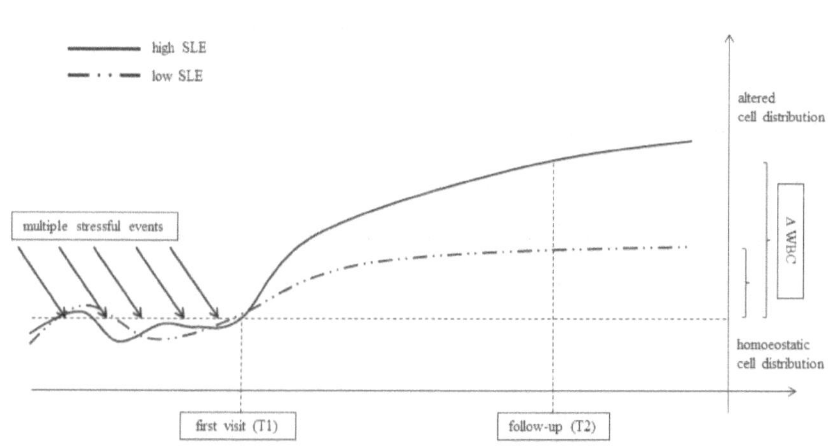

Figure 7. Basic research model explaining the change in white blood cells due to life stress. *Note:* SLE = stressful life events, WBC = white blood cells (neutrophils, lymphocytes, monocytes), ΔWBC = WBCT2 − WBCT1. It is hypothesized that glucocorticoids have a systematic modulating effect on the distribution of WBC at all stages depicted in the figure.

7.3   Material and methods

7.3.1   *Study population*

The current study included participants from the ongoing prospective Dresden Burnout Study (DBS; Penz, Wekenborg et al., 2018) that was conducted in accordance with the Declaration of Helsinki and therefore approved by the local ethics committee. DBS participants were recruited Germany-wide through public media platforms and the civil register of the city Dresden. Inclusion criterion was restricted to working age (between 18 and 68) and language (sufficient language skills to fill out German questionnaires). All the DBS participants residing in Dresden and within a 60 km radius of the city were invited for the assessment of biological markers. The DBS was conducted with an emphasis on the city and region of Dresden, which contributed approx. one -third to the whole sample. 1.864 participants were invited for the first visit of biomarker sampling that was conducted from September to October 2015, out of which 446 accepted our invitation. 2.795 participants were invited for the second visit (857 recruited by the Dresden civil register), resulting in data from 507 participants at visit two. The second study wave was conducted from October to November 2016 and from January to February 2017. Altogether, 173 participants attended both, study visit one (T1) and study visit two (T2; first follow up), representing the current longitudinal study sample. Due to unsuccessful blood sampling at T1 and/or T2, longitudinal WBC data were available only from 154 participants (mean ± SD age at T1: 42.16 ± 11.74; 67.5% female). Detailed sample characteristics for T1 and T2 are summarized in Table 5. All the participants received a monetary reward of 15 euros on T1 and T2.

7.3.2   *Materials and methods*

One week prior to the laboratory session, the participants completed questionnaires including the MBI-GS (Büssing & Glaser, 1999) and the PHQ-9 (Löwe et al., 2002) together with information about sociodemographic and health-related factors as well as about hair treatment (summarized in Table 5). Laboratory sessions were conducted between 7 am and 7 pm with an average duration of 50 minutes. The session included a blood draw, hair sample collection, assessment of the HRV (T1 data reported by Kanthak et al., 2017), and assessment of the Life Stressor Checklist (LSC-R). EDTA-whole blood samples were stored at room temperature for a maximum of five hours and then transferred to a medical laboratory (Medizinisches Labor Ostsachsen, Dresden) for WBC subset analyses (percent neutrophils, lymphocytes, and monocytes). Hair strands were cut as close as possible to the scalp from a posterior vertex position. The first three centimetres most proximal to the scalp were analyzed, which represents a marker for the cumulative GC secretion 3 months prior to sampling (given an average hair growth of 1 cm per month; Wennig, 2000). The shampooing procedure and the GC extraction were conducted as described in the laboratory protocol by Gao et al. (2013) and analyzed by liquid chromatography coupled with tandem mass spectrometry (LC-MS/MS).

Table 5: Sample characteristics for baseline and follow-up.

	T1 (N = 417)		T2 (N = 154)	
	M (SD)	*Range*	*M (SD)*	*Range*
Demographics				
Age (year)	41.3 (11.2)	18 – 66	42.2 (11.7)	21 – 66
Female (%)	65.5		67.5	
Body mass index (kg/m^2)	25.1 (4.4)	17.3 – 41.8	24.9 (4.1)	15.2 – 37.5
Smokers (%)	12.5		11.5	
Health-related variables				
LSC-R sum score	3.3 (3.8)	0 – 19	3.4 (3.8)	0 – 15
LSC-R$_{CIS}$	14.3 (11.8)	1 – 90	14.2 (12.3)	1 – 90
MBI-GS total score	2.2 (1.1)	0 – 5.4	2.2 (1.2)	0 – 4.5
PHQ-9 sum score	8.3 (5.3)	0 – 26	7.8 (4.9)	0 – 23
Hair characteristics				
Washes per week	3.5 (1.8)	1 – 7	3.3 (1.8)	1 – 7
Coloration %	31.4		28.6	

Note. Standard deviations are in parentheses. LSC-R = Life Stressor Checklist – Revised; LSC-R$_{CIS}$ = LSC-R cumulative impact score; MBI-GS = Maslach Burnout Inventory - General Survey; PHQ-9 = Patient Health Questionnaire

7.3.3 *Assessment of stressful life events*

During the baseline assessment, participants completed the Life Stressor Checklist-Revised (LSC-R; Wolfe, Kimerling, Brown, Chrestman, & Levin, 1996) for the assessment of cumulative stressful events over the life- span. The LSC-R is a 30-item self-report measure with good psychometric properties (test-retest reliability κ for all subscales between 0.51 and 0.76 for a 7-days-interval; McHugo et al., 2005). The items represent SLE that meet the criteria for a traumatic event or are considered as highly stressful experiences (Hathaway, Boals, & Banks, 2010; McHugo et al., 2005). All the items can be answered in a yes/no format. In case of a `yes´-answer, a Likert scale from 1 (not at all) to 5 (extreme) represents how much the certain event influenced the precedent year. The total number of the different event types experienced can be determined by summing up the `yes´-answers (Humphreys et al., 2011). To weight these reported SLE by their subjective relevance (e.g. the unexpected death of a participant's great-grandfather during his/her childhood may not necessarily impact on the current life situation anymore), the SLE measure was calculated by summing the 5-point Likert scale items, representing the cumulative impact of the SLE (LSC-R cumulative impact scale; LSC-R$_{CIS}$) during the year prior to assessment, resulting in scores ranging from 0 to 150 (Choi, Kim, Jang, Bae, & Kim, 2017). Accordingly, the LSC-R$_{CIS}$ served as primary indicator of SLE as it does not just summarize the amount of SLE a person experienced over the life -span, but represents a measure of how affected the person felt by the reported cumulative SLE during the 12 months prior to assessment.

7.3.4 *Data processing and statistical analyses*

Based on the log-normal distribution model, we removed extreme manifestations of HCC and WBC percentages ($\pm$ 3 standard deviations from the mean of the log-scaled outcomes) in a first step, leaving a total of n = 148 participants who provided WBC data at baseline and follow-up. Supplementary HCC analyses were conducted based on a subsample of N = 104 participants.

Primary analyses: Three linear regression analyses were conducted to estimate the predictive value of LSC-R_{CIS} on the temporal change of different leukocyte subsets (X: percent neutrophils, N_{eut}; lymphocytes, L_{ym}; monocytes, M_{ono}). The relative change of these leukocyte subsets from T1 to T2 was modelled as follows:

$$\Delta X = \log(X_{T2}) - \log(X_{T1}) = \log(X_{T2}/X_{T1})$$

Regression coefficients were estimated using the following linear predictor:

$$\text{model 1: } \Delta X = \beta_0 + \beta_1 * \log(X_{T1}) + \beta_2 * \text{LSC-}R_{CIS} + \varepsilon$$

β_0 = intercept; β_1 = regression coefficient for log(X) at T1; β_2 = regression coefficient for LSC-R_{CIS} (scale: 10 pts). This modelling procedure allows for attributing the impact of all time-invariant confounders to β_1 (e.g. sex, age, physical predispositions), which yields a tremendously increased statistical power to detect even small effects of SLE via β_2. Multiple testing was accounted for by the Bonferroni adjustment, resulting in a significance threshold of $p < \alpha = 1.67\%$ to maintain a family-wise error rate of 5%.

Secondary analyses: Based on model 1, model 2 was fitted to estimate the predictive value of LSC-R_{CIS} on the N_{eut}/L_{ym} ratio at T2:

$$\text{model 2: } \log(\text{ratio}) = \beta_0 + \beta_1 * \log(N_{eutT1}) + \beta_2 * \log(L_{ymT1}) + \beta_3 * \text{LSC-}R_{CIS} + \varepsilon$$

β_0 = intercept; β_1 = regression coefficient for $\log(N_{eut})$ at T1; β_2 = regression coefficient for $\log(L_{ym})$ at T1; β_3 = regression coefficient for LSC-R_{CIS}.

In three further analyses, we estimated the association between concurrent changes in HCC and X (N_{eut}, L_{ym}, and M_{ono}). Relative changes in HCC were modelled analogously to model 1:

$$\Delta HCC = \log(HCC_{T2}) - \log(HCC_{T1}) = \log(HCC_{T2}/HCC_{T1})$$

Regression coefficients were estimated using the extended linear predictor:

$$\text{model 3: } \Delta X = \beta_0 + \beta_1 * \log(X_{T1}) + \beta_2 * \text{LSC-}R_{CIS} + \beta_3 * \Delta HCC + \varepsilon$$

with β_0 = intercept; β_1 = regression coefficient for X at T1; β_2 = regression coefficient for LSC-RCIS; β_3 = regression coefficient for change in HCC.

We further checked for additional variance explained by interaction and/or primary effects of SLE and HCC (visualized in Figure 8). Based on this model, we investigated the incremental portion of variance explained by HCC and its interaction with SLE.

As neither burnout nor depression was part of the current research agenda, the assessed instruments (MBI-GS and PHQ-9) were not considered for our methods section.

7.4   Results

Table 6 shows WBC compositions (i.e. the different leukocyte subsets) and HCC at T1 and T2. Regression coefficients for the main and the additional analysis are reported in Table 7.

Table 6: Blood and hair characteristics from the longitudinal sample (N = 154).

| | T1 | | T2 | |
	M (SD)	*Range*	*M (SD)*	*Range*
Blood				
Leukocytes (Gpt/l)	6.6 (1.7)	3.2 – 14.5	6.2 (1.5)	3.6 – 13.1
Neutrophils (%)	56.6 (8.2)	38.8 – 78.2	52.4 (9.3)	29.5 – 74.4
Lymphocytes (%)	31.8 (7.3)	12.4 – 49.4	34.4 (8.8)	3.5 – 57.5
Monocytes (%)	8.0 (1.9)	3.5 – 15.2	9.2 (3.7)	3.4 – 46.6
Hair (N = 114)				
HCC (pg/mg)	14.9 (13.5)	0.4 – 60.3	6.2 (4.0)	0.1 – 21.5

Note. Standard deviations are in parentheses; HCC = hair cortisol concentrations

Primary analyses: There was a significant effect of LSC-R$_{CIS}$ in the relative change of N$_{eut}$ between T1 and T2 (R^2 = 0.21, $F_{(2,148)}$ = 20.13, p = 0.01), suggesting a mean increase of ΔN$_{eut}$ from T1 to T2 with a factor of 1.027 (2.8%) per 10 points LSC-R$_{CIS}$. The maximum observed LSC-R$_{CIS}$ of 80 points was predicted to increase the relative change in N$_{eut}$ by approx. 31% as compared to the reference change in N$_{eut}$ at 0 points LSC-R$_{CIS}$ (see Figure 8). Under these reference conditions, the relative change in N$_{eut}$ from T1 to T2 decreased on average by -10.6%. Accordingly, we observed a significant attenuation of the overall decrease in N_{eut} due to cumulative life stress. An effect of LSC-R_{CIS} on relative change of L_{ym} was indicated as a trend and points to a 3.2% mean decline of lymphocytes per 10 points LSC-R_{CIS}. In other words, with each 10 points on the LSC-R_{CIS}, ΔL_{ym} decreased from T1 to T2 by -3.2%. However, the regression coefficient for LSC-R_{CIS} did not fall below the Bonferroni-adjusted significance level ($R^2 = 0.32$, $F_{(2,148)} = 34.96$, $p = 0.04$). Under reference conditions with 0 points in the LSC-R_{CIS}, L_{ym} increased with a factor of 1.128 (12.8%). Each 10 points LSC-R_{CIS} attenuated this increase in L_{ym} by -3.2%. There was no robust effect of LSC-R_{CIS} on the change of monocytes ($R^2 = 0.16$, $F_{(2,148)} = 13.93$, $p = 0.71$).

Table 7: Regression coefficients for main and additional analyses.

	β_0	β_1	β_2	β_3
Model[1]: LSC-R_{CIS}				
ΔN_{eut} (%)	-0.11 (0.02)**	-0.07 (0.01)**	0.03 (0.01)*	
ΔL_{ym} (%)	0.12 (0.03)**	-0.15 (0.02)**	-0.03 (0.02)°	
ΔM_{ono} (%)	0.11 (0.02)**	-0.07 (0.01)**	> 0.01 (0.01)	
Model[2]: LSC-R_{CIS}				
Δ ratio (%)	0.38 (0.05)**	0.08 (0.06)	-0.08 (0.07)	0.06 (0.03)*
Model[3]:HCC				
ΔN_{eut} (%)	-0.10 (0.03)**	-0.07 (0.01)**	0.04 (0.02)*	0.03 (0.01)*
ΔL_{ym} (%)	-0.10 (0.04)*	-0.15 (0.02)**	-0.04 (0.02)	-0.04 (0.02)*
ΔM_{ono} (%)	0.08 (0.02)**	-0.06 (0.01)**	> 0.01 (0.01)	-0.04 (0.01)**

Note: N_{eut} = neutrophils; L_{ym} = lymphocytes; M_{ono} = monocytes; ratio = N_{eut}/L_{ym}; LSC-R_{CIS} = Life Stressor checklist cumulative impact scale; HCC = hair cortisol concentrations; Model[1]: **p < 0.001, *p < 0.016, °p < 0.05; Model[1]/Model[2]: **p < 0.01, *p < 0.05

Secondary analysis:

<u>Neutrophil-to-Lymphocyte ratio:</u> There was suggestive evidence for an effect of LSC-R_{CIS} on the N_{eut}/L_{ym} ratio at T2 ($R^2 = 0.18$, $F_{(3,147)} = 10.49$, $p = 0.02$) that manifested as an increase of 6.2% per 10 points LSC-R_{CIS}. Under reference conditions (i.e. at 0 points LSC-R_{CIS}) the mean N_{eut}/L_{ym} ratio amounted to 1.46 (i.e., the portion of N_{eut} was 46% higher than those of L_{ym} at T2).

<u>Hair cortisol concentrations:</u> Change in HCC suggestively predicted the relative change of all WBC subsets (ΔN_{eut}: $\beta_{\Delta HCC} = 0.03$, $p = 0.03$, $\Delta R^2 = 0.05$; ΔL_{ym}: $\beta_{\Delta HCC} = -0.04$, $p = 0.02$, $\Delta R^2 = 0.04$; ΔM_{ono}: $\beta_{\Delta HCC} = -0.04$, $p < 0.01$, $\Delta R^2 = 0.07$). N_{eut} increased with a factor of 1.029 (2.9%), L_{ym} decreased with a factor of 0.957 (4.3%), and M_{ono} decreased with a factor of 0.964 (3.6%) across the interquartile range of the ΔHCC.

<u>Interactions between SLE and HCC:</u> There is a tentative effect of SLE on the interaction between ΔHCC and ΔN_{eut} [$RSS = 2.74$, $F_{(2,103)} = 3.55$, $p = 0.03$] and on the interaction between ΔHCC and ΔL_{ym} [$RSS = 6.05$, $F_{(2,103)} = 3.67$, $p = 0.03$]. On the contrary, there is no effect of SLE on the interaction between ΔHCC and ΔM_{ono}. Results are depicted in Figure 8.

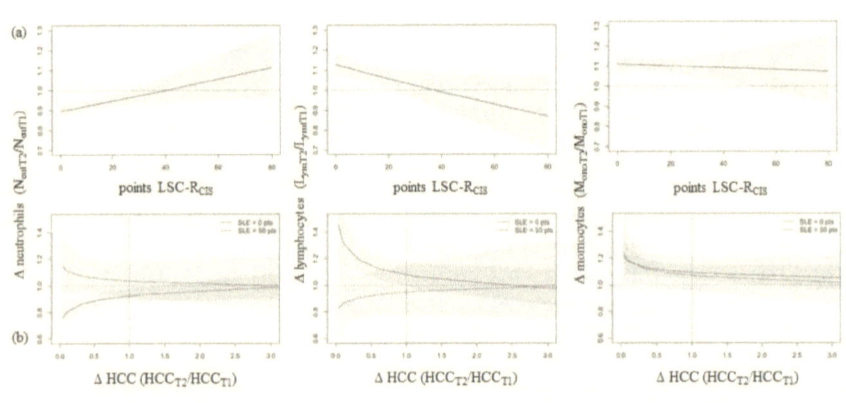

Figure 8. Model summary for primary analyses (a) and for analyses of main and interactional effects (b). *Note:* Δ = value T2 – value T1, LSC-RCIS = Life Stressor Checklist revised (cumulative impact scale) , HCC = hair cortisol concentrations, SLE = stressful life events

7.5 Discussion

The present study assessed the impact of cumulative SLE on the change of WBCs (neutrophils, lymphocytes, and monocytes) within one year. It further gives insight into one potential factor that may account for leukocyte distribution in peripheral blood, namely GCs (measured with HCC). Our data suggest an attenuation of the overall decrease (synonymic with an increase) of neutrophils from first visit (T1) to one year follow-up (T2) due to the impact of SLE prior to T1 (life stressor checklist cumulative impact scale; LSC-R_{CIS}). This differential one-year change in neutrophils was more pronounced when HCC concurrently increased across the investigated follow-up period, which suggests a systematic effect of GCs on neutrophil distribution. These results are in line with previous animal (Dhabhar et al., 2012; Dhabhar & Mcewen, 1997) and human (Cole, 2008; McKinnon et al., 1989; Miller et al., 2005) data, suggesting that one path on which (psychological) stress enters the body is at the level of leukocyte distribution in peripheral blood. This is also in line with the hypothesis that the peripheral distribution of leukocytes is to a detectable extent regulated by GCs (Cohen et al., 2012). In our study, each 10 point increase in LSC-R_{CIS} was associated with a 2.8% increase in the one-year neutrophils change, which resulted in a maximum increase of 31% (80 LSC-R_{CIS} points). By comparison, Dhabhar et al. (2012) found a 75% increase in neutrophils 120 min after stress exposure. In contrast to the attenuated decrease in neutrophils, we found an attenuated increase (synonymic with decrease) in lymphocytes due to SLE, which is likewise comparable with rodent data by Dhabhar et al. (2012) and Engler et al. (2004). In our study, the lymphocyte change decreased by -3.2% per 10 points LSC-R_{CIS}, which did not fall below the Bonferroni-adjusted significance threshold but was still indicated as a trend. Data on bone marrow leukopoiesis in response to immune activation suggests a reciprocal effect for neutrophils and lymphocytes (Ueda et al., 2005). Assumed that SLE triggered an immune response in our sample that would be in line with an increase in neutrophils change and a simultaneous decrease in lymphocytes change as here observed. Opposed to Engler et al. (2004), but in line with Dhabhar et al. (2012), we found no significant change in monocytes, suggesting that monocytes did not alter in response to the cumulative SLE in our sample.

To our knowledge, there is no other human data available that assessed the GC-driven kinetics of WBCs in response to SLE in a time window of several months. Animal data by Engler et al. (2004) and Dhabhar et al. (2012) used stressors with a clearly definable stress on- and offset. Blood counts were taken immediately after (cumulative) stress exposure and were analyzed in relation to non-stressed control subjects. Data on potential long-term stress-related alterations in human WBCs have been missing so far , but cross-sectional data consistently support a theory of maladaptive immune alterations as a consequence of chronic stress (discussed in Cohen et al., 2007; Dhabhar, 2014; Glaser & Kiecolt-Glaser, 2005). This theory probably also generalizes the type of stress exposure indicated by the SLE. Cohen and colleagues (2012), for example, showed that exposure to a recent major life event significantly increases the risk for developing a cold after exposure to a rhino virus.

It might be assumed that exposure to SLE initially provokes an immune enhancement which, in the long run, leads to maladaptive alterations if the stressor is somehow ongoing. We hypothesize that repetitive life stress might heighten the psychological and immunological alertness of an individual and that the initial protective enhancement of immune defense in expectation of a stressful event triggers maladaptive processes (Dhabhar, 2014), e.g., chronic inflammation (Rohleder, 2012, 2014). An increased neutrophil production, for example, could be interpreted as a protective compensatory mechanism to replenish cells lost through an immune response, since activated granulocytes are unable to divide and survive only for a couple of hours (Ueda et al., 2004). One might speculate that an initial stress-induced up-regulation of neutrophils in the periphery represents a direct source of chronic inflammatory processes. Neutrophils are not just essential for host defense and tissue healing, they also induce a highly toxic environment, are important sources of pro-inflammatory cytokines (e.g. tumour necrosis factor, TNF), and are involved in the pathology of various inflammatory conditions (Nathan, 2006; Scapini & Cassatella, 2014; Smith, 1994). If an initial increase in neutrophils generates an inflammatory process, inflammation could in turn act as a signal to recruit even more neutrophils to damaged target tissues, initiating a vicious circle of immune defense, tissue damage, and systemic inflammation which would not be expected in the absence of a trigger (SLE). For a further exploration of the hypotheses for neutrophil-related inflammation, future studies should simultaneously assess leukocyte subsets, HCC, and inflammation markers (e.g. CRP, TNF-α; Rohleder, 2014).

7.5.1 *Hair cortisol concentration and glucocorticoid resistance*

Our study design additionally provides HCC data to assess if a change in WBCs in response to SLE is associated with the change in GCs between T1 and T2. Each interquartile increase in HCC from T1 to T2 tentatively predicted a 2.9% increase in the neutrophil change, a 4.3% decrease in lymphocyte change, and a 3.6% decrease in monocyte change. GCs are known to have down-regulatory effects on the production of several chemokines and chemoattractants that curb leukocyte migration (Cain & Cidlowski, 2017) and have previously been described as having immune-suppressive properties (Glaser and Kiecolt-Glaser, 2005; Dhabhar, 2014). A tentative dampening effect of cortisol on lymphocyte and monocyte distribution as suggested by our data is in line with Dhabhar et al. (2012) who showed a significant effect for lymphocytes and monocytes but not for neutrophils after hormone treatment. Interestingly, in our data, neutrophils were tentatively associated with HCC but the direction suggests a GC-driven upregulation of neutrophils. These results, however, are based on exploratory analyses and therefore need to be confirmed by future studies that are specifically designed to investigate the GC-driven kinetics of neutrophils compared to lymphocytes and monocytes. It further surprises that a change in monocytes may also be associated with a relative change in HCC independent of SLE.

Our study supports the theory that GCs are key molecules for the distribution of WBCs, as hypothesized in the glucocorticoid resistance (GCR) model (Miller et al., 2002; Pariante, 2017). The GCR model supposes that chronic stress diminishes the immune system's sensitivity to GCs as a consequence of a counter-regulatory response to an initial GC overexposure (Miller et al., 2002). Consequently, any GCR following SLE exposure is supposed to result in attenuated associations between WBCs and GCs (Cohen et al., 2012). In our overall sample we found tentative associations between the change in HCC and WBCs. As depicted in Figure 8, exposure to SLE changed the effect of HCC on neutrophils and lymphocytes (not on monocytes). The increase of neutrophils and decrease of lymphocytes that could be observed under the reference condition (0 pts LSC-R_{CIS}) seemed to reverse under the influence of life stress (SLE). Even if conclusions must be interpreted carefully and are based on the presumptions that the model is correct, our data can be interpreted in line with GCR as, for instance, shown by Cole (2008). It should also be considered by future studies that a WBC and GC interaction may develop in different stages, with an initial systematic reciprocity that exclusively leads to a total dissolution between stress and the immune system at a very chronic stage.

7.5.2 *Neutrophil-to-Lymphocyte ratio*

Regarding shared variance between neutrophils and lymphocytes and reciprocal leukopoiesis in bone marrow (Ueda et al., 2005; Ueda et al., 2004), we additionally investigated the neutrophil/lymphocyte ratio by further exploratory analyses. The neutrophil/lymphocyte ratio was tentatively predicted by the psychological stress due to SLE the year before T1 (LSC-R_{CIS}). The ratio increased with a factor of 6.2% per LSC-R_{CIS} unit (10 points). This is in line with cross-sectional data by Cole (2008) who found the neutrophil/lymphocyte ratio to be particularly sensitive to physiologic variations in endogenous cortisol and associated with stressful life experience (loneliness).

Taken together, our data suggest considerable long-term alterations in neutrophils and lymphocytes resulting in a joint change of the neutrophil/lymphocyte ratio due to the impact of temporally preceding SLE. The change in monocytes was independent of SLE. The change of neutrophils, lymphocytes, and monocytes was further associated with the available amount of the GCs. Although the longitudinal design perfectly controls for stable, inter-individual confounders and, thus, yields increased power to detect effects as compared to cross-sectional designs, our study shows some shortcomings and limitations. First, the reported findings are based on a sample with high prevalence of burnout symptomatology. Thus, the SLE variability might have been larger than compared to the general population, which in turn may have increased the probability of detecting small effects that are negligible from a clinical perspective. Second, the LSC-R was only assessed during the Dresden Burnout Study baseline assessment as additional information. There is no information about experience or impact of subsequent SLE in the year between T1 and T2, which apparently might also contribute to the change of WBCs and GC levels. In this regard, a continuous monitoring of SLEs across time might provide more detailed information. Further, the LSC-R$_{CIS}$ provides an estimate of the total amount and latest relevance of SLE. Information on the time interval between experiencing a certain event and the baseline is missing. It might contribute to the psychological and immunological effects whether, for instance, the reported event was experienced in childhood/adolescence or happened recently. For a more detailed exploration of the time-dependent effects of SLE, childhood trauma should be included in further assessments. Indeed, adverse childhood experiences were included as part of the LSC-R$_{CIS}$ but could not be analyzed separately from the later SLE, which does not allow for any conclusion on a potential time window for the reported effects in WBCs and GC levels. Accordingly, future studies should consider the existence of temporally varying effects by assessing immunological alterations at shorter time intervals (Dorman & Griffin, 2015), for instance, with consecutive monthly assessments of the WBCs and GCs. The future aim should be a description of the kinetics in cells and molecules (e.g. hormones, cytokines, and proteins) that mediate an immune response, to provide elaborated understanding of the path between life stress experiences and disease. Most certainly, for a correct interpretation of the results it must be taken into consideration that the present study was conducted to solely evaluate the long-term influence of the SLE on leukocytes subsets as marginal effects. Information about other potential time-dependent mediators is missing. For instance, it can be concluded that a person with an adverse experience caused by SLE may also score high on other clinical relevant features, e.g., burnout or depression. Further, measurement bias has to be considered as mood states like burnout or depression might influence the probability of reporting particular items (Lavoie & Douglas, 2012). Also other intra-individual variables (e.g. genetics and epigenetics) might contribute significantly to the patterns between SLE, leukocyte subsets, and HCC. Despite these shortcomings, the current results provide a sound basis for supporting the assumption that adverse life experience enters the body by maladaptive alterations at the immune level, which as a consequence might increase the vulnerability for negative health outcomes over the whole life-span.

8 General discussion

After a brief review of the underlying theoretical assumptions of this book, main and additional results from Study 1 and Study 2 will be discussed based on the following aims:

i. Assessment of the endocrine stress response (HCC) due to chronic stress exposure (burnout).

ii. Assessment of a one-year immune response (distribution of leukocyte differentials) due to chronic stress exposure (SLE).

iii. Assessment of a long-term (1 year) interaction between the HCC and leukocyte distribution under the influence of chronic stress exposure (SLE).

iv. Integration of results into the extended version of the stage model by Cohen and colleagues (2016; Figure 4).

8.1 Brief summary of the general research model

Chronic stress exposure has been reported as a risk factor for several adverse health conditions, for instance, atherothrombotic (Austin et al., 2013), autoimmune (Porcelli et al., 2016), and/or cardiovascular (Dimsdale, 2008; Golbidi et al., 2015) diseases. Increased disease vulnerability as a consequence of chronic stress exposure is hypothesized to be due to long-lasting alterations in the activation of *allostatic* systems, such as the HPA axis and the immune system. Potentially health-challenging alterations are named *allostatic load/overload* and represent the 'costs' of adapting to a long-term stress exposure (McEwen, 1998a, 1998b; Cohen & Wingfield, 2003).

The HPA axis regulates the availability of GC hormones such as cortisol (Tsigos & Chrousos, 2002). Virtually all immune cells provide receptors for GC hormones that can modulate immune cell functions through binding to these receptors (e.g. GRs/MRs; Glaser &

Kiecolt-Glaser, 2005). An interplay between the HPA axis and the immune system in adaptive stress has been described by several theoretical models with the aim of explaining the health- challenging effects of chronic stress exposure (e.g. Chrousos, 2009; Elenkov & Chrousos, 2006; Glaser & Kiecolt-Glaser, 2005; Shields & Slavich, 2017). Notably, human studies exploring the interplay between the HPA axis and the leukocyte differentials in response to stress exposure have been scarce so far. This book aims at closing the gap by the exploration of cortisol, leukocyte differentials, and their interaction in response to work overload and cumulative SLE.

8.2 Chronic stress exposure related to burnout and the HPA axis stress response

Study 1 aimed the cross-sectional assessment of potential HPA axis alterations due to chronic stress exposure by burnout. Additionally, for a broader exploration, data from Study 2 was considered as well for the general discussion. The endocrine stress response in Study 1 was defined as significant burnout-associated change in the availability of free cortisol measured with HCC. The result of this book supports a hypothesis of elevated cortisol levels in burnout sufferers. Notably, just the dichotomized burnout marker showed associations, whereas a continuous burnout score was unrelated to HCC.

For a generalized interpretation it must be considered that Study 1 was the first to assess cortisol in burnout sufferers on the basis of HCC, whereas previous studies used single time point measures of cortisol (from saliva, serum, and urinary). Single time point measures are more susceptible to daily fluctuations than HCC (Russell et al., 2012) and reflect acute rather than long-term cortisol levels (Sauvé et al., 2007). A direct comparison might therefore be misleading. Notably, results based on single time point measures showed mixed outcomes and indicated both up- or downregulation of available cortisol as well as no associations (systematic review and analysis: Danhof-Pont et al., 2011). Oosterholt and colleagues (2015), for example, showed a lower cortisol awakening response (CAR) in burnout sufferers compared to healthy controls and concluded burnout to be associated with a hypoactive HPA axis. Likewise, Marchand et al. (2014) and Juster et al. (2011) found support for a blunted HPA axis and lowered overall cortisol levels. Interestingly, data by Wingenfeld, Schulz, Damkroeger, Rose, and Driessen (2009) found the circadian cortisol cycle (CAR) unrelated to burnout symptomatology, but the overall daily cortisol suggested a hyperactive HPA axis with raised cortisol levels.

Herr et al. (2018) published data on work stress and HCC which provides important information for the discussion of results from Study 1. Indeed, comparability to Study 1 (Penz, Stalder et al., 2018) is restricted by the fact that work stress was defined on the basis of effort reward imbalance (ERI). Differing from the results in Study 1, Herr et al. (2018) found no significant cross-sectional associations between work stress and HCC but showed a positive long-term association for the course of one year. Even if the sample was small and solely included male participants, these data support a hypothesis of elevated HCC in people suffering from chronic stress at work. In contrast to Herr et al. (2018), additional information about HCC from baseline and follow-up provided by Study 2 fails to replicate the long-term associations between burnout and HCC. Neither was burnout experienced the months before baseline assessment associated with a change in HCC between baseline and follow-up nor was a one-year change in burnout symptomatology associated with the change in HCC (additional analyses, not reported in paper 3).

8.2.1 *Exhaustion versus work overload: different definitions of burnout*

Besides the difference in specimens, study designs exploring the HPA axis activation in burnout sufferers partly differ in relation to the underlying burnout definitions. It is tempting to speculate that a respective definition of burnout and its symptomatology contribute to characteristics of the adaptive stress response (e.g. by defining the duration of stress exposure) and might therefore account for the heterogeneity in the results. Chida and Steptoe (2009) provide meta-analytic support for an increased CAR in association with job stress. Job stress might be speculated to be an obligatory characteristic in burnout. On the other hand, in the same meta-analysis, Chida and Steptoe (2009) showed that burnout (classed together with fatigue or exhaustion) was associated with a reduced CAR. Even if these results seem contradictory at first sight, the discrepancies might result from differences in the definition of burnout/fatigue. Maslach et al. (2001), for instance, consider 'exhaustion' the most obvious manifestation of burnout. If exhaustion is central in the definition of burnout symptomatology, the concept shares the main characteristics with CFS (Huibers et al., 2003; Leone et al., 2011) which is commonly associated with a blunted HPA axis activity and decreased cortisol levels (Afari & Buchwald, 2014). The symptomatology of CFS (e.g. sleep disturbances, reduced physical activity) is even speculated to be a consequence of down-regulated cortisol levels, which is supported by the fact that replacement therapy with synthetic cortisol (hydrocortisone) improves CFS symptoms (discussed in Cleare, 2004). In analogy to CFS, alterations at the level of the HPA axis might be considered a risk factor for the burnout symptom 'exhaustion'. Established burnout questionnaires are based on a burnout definition that understands 'exhaustion' as central in the symptomatology of the syndrome, shown for instance by the MBI-GS (Maslach et al., 2001), the Oldenburg Burnout Inventory (Halbesleben & Demerouti, 2005), the Shirom-Melamed-Burnout Measure (Shirom & Melamed, 2006), and the Copenhagen Burnout Inventory (Kristensen et al., 2005). In contrast, instruments that operationalize work stress outside the context of burnout, such as the ERI (Siegrist et al., 2004; Siegrist, Wege, Pühlhofer, & Wahrendorf, 2009), assess the appraisal of work stress and work overload. It seems reasonable to speculate that cortisol acts as a burnout risk factor by modulating burnout symptoms such as 'energy loss' or 'feeling of fatigue'. This hypothesis might explain negative associations between cortisol and burnout symptomatology in case burnout is defined as a syndrome of exhaustion. Future research projects should explore if altered cortisol levels represent a risk factor for developing a burnout syndrome. Heim et al. (2009), for instance, showed that childhood trauma and a trauma-associated blunted HPA axis activity is a significant risk factor for developing CFS. Comparative associations might be speculated for the progression of burnout.

In contrast, increased cortisol levels in people who report a high level of stress and work load (e.g. as measured by the ERI questionnaire; Herr et al., 2018), might represent an initial physiological coping mechanism for maintaining *allostasis* in a stressful work situation. Due to the physiological effects of cortisol, a long -term up-regulation of its availability might support an individual in facing the stress situation at work, for instance, by energy supply (Sapolsky et al., 2000) and increased attention (Tsigos & Chrousos, 2002). In case of chronic/long-term stress exposure and/or prior charge by antecedent stress exposure (e.g. childhood trauma), counter-regulatory mechanisms may interfere and change the pattern from up- to down-regulation of cortisol and/or cortisol action (Figures 2 and 3).

8.3   <u>Chronic stress exposure and the distribution of leukocyte differentials</u>

Study 2 was aimed at examining the effect of stress exposure due to SLE on the peripheral distribution of leukocyte differentials (neutrophils, lymphocytes, monocytes). In line with the research hypothesis of this book (Figures 1-3), our results suggest that chronic stress exposure manifests in alterations at the level of the immune system. Manifestations were shown for the peripheral distribution of neutrophils, as well as tentatively suggested for lymphocytes. Study 2 was designed to explore long-term disease-related alterations due to chronic stress exposure. Considering that leukocyte differentials contribute to the immune defense and host protection (Dhabhar, 2014; Segerstrom & Miller, 2004; Smith, 1994), our data suggest a potential pathway for the transmission from a phenomenon of the mind (appraisal of a stressor; Figure 4) via increased vulnerability to adverse health conditions. This also suggests that alterations at the level of the immune system can stay in the body for several months or even years after stress cessation. A continuous increase in neutrophils can be substantiated by study data from a second follow-up two years after the assessment of the SLE (third visit of DBS biomarker sampling; data in preparation for publication). The second follow-up provides longitudinal blood data (leukocyte differentials) from 124 participants (mean ± SD age at T3: 44.10 ± 11.72; 72.10% female). Using the same statistical models as reported in Study 2, the peripheral distribution of neutrophils still tended to show an increase if participants reported a high number of SLE during the baseline assessment two years earlier ($R^2 = 0.26$, $F_{(1,115)} = 20.22$, $p = 0.06$), which strengthens the research model of Study 2 (specified for the peripheral distribution of neutrophils; Figure 7). The trend suggested for a stress-related decrease in lymphocytes reported in Study 2 disappeared in the time frame of two years.

Notably, the generalizability of results is restricted by certain characteristics of the design of Study 2, especially to the type of stress exposure. It might be speculated that exposure to cumulative SLE differs from other chronic stressors (e.g. loneliness, burnout) insofar that the assessed stress is based on events experienced throughout the life- span. The reported stress experience can likewise include distant events (e.g. childhood maltreatment) as well as recent stress experiences. Also, Study 2 assessed SLE without distinction between stress exposure due to a single traumatic experience (e.g. car accident) and chronic stress exposure, such as suffering from a severe mental or physical disease (Wolfe et al., 1996).

Despite these restrictions, the long-term association between the neutrophils and the SLE shown by Study 2 suggest a stable and remarkable immune alteration that is interpreted as adaptive immune response to the chronic exposure to life stress. Importantly, it needs to be noted that not the sum of experienced events was associated with neutrophil distribution (and tentatively indicated for lymphocytes), but the appraisal of how much impact these events had on people's lives within the year prior to baseline assessment. Interestingly, the 'objective' sum of all reported SLE over the course of the life- span did not show any associations with leukocyte differentials (additional analyses, not reported in study 2).

It seems reasonable to conclude that stress experience due to SLE can cause a long-term stress response, either because the event itself is ongoing or because psychological consequences of the event. (e.g., negative emotional response) are ongoing. Considering the stage model of stress and disease by Cohen and colleagues (2016; Figure 4), a stressful event (e.g., watching a lethal car accident; level 1, Figure 4) is potentially health-challenging via the above discussed pathways (Figures 1-3), given that it is appraised as stressful at the moment of its occurrence (level 2, Figure 4). Long-term alterations at the level of the immune system (e.g. continuous rise of peripheral neutrophils; level 5) due to SLE might be expected if the event is still experienced as stressful in a retrospective evaluation, causing an ongoing negative emotional response (level 3). Under these conditions it can be speculated that the endocrine and immunological (levels 4 and 5) stress responses are also ongoing, increasing the vulnerability to adverse health conditions (level 6) in the long term (Figures 2 and 3). Long-term stress-related alterations that precede an adverse health condition can be hypothesized as a continuous process (Figure 7) that proceeds as long as the stress experience is ongoing. Further, a dose-response relation between the severity of the stress experience and the *allostatic load/overload* can be assumed, as it was shown, for instance, by Danese, Pariante, Caspi, Taylor, and Poulton (2007) for associations between childhood maltreatment and inflammation.

8.4   Long-term interactions between HPA axis and leukocyte differentials

The research model of this book is based on the hypothesis that stress experience enters the body at the level of the HPA axis, which was supported by Study 1. Cortisol as the main effector of the HPA axis (Tsigos & Chrousos, 2002) was assumed further to interact with the immune system that in return modulates the activity of the HPA axis (Glaser & Kiecolt-Glaser, 2005). Considering a bidirectional interaction between the HPA axis and the immune system, it seems reasonable to hypothesize that alterations due to stress exposure are found within both physiological systems in parallel. Study 2 additionally tested such an interactional progression (Figure 8). Our data indicate that the change in HCC between baseline and follow-up was associated with the one-year change in the distribution of the leukocyte subsets, which supports the theory of an interactional progression. Surprisingly, associations were most pronounced for monocytes, although the one-year change in monocyte distribution was independent of the SLE.

A priori assumptions for the interaction between cortisol and leukocyte differentials were ambiguous. On the one hand, a correlational relationship between the one-year change in HCC and the one-year change in leukocyte distribution was expected, indicating that alterations in the amount of circulating cortisol modulate the distribution of leukocyte differentials and vice versa. On the other hand, hypotheses in Study 2 were based on the idea of GCR. GCR represents a condition of insufficient GC signalling due to insensitive GRs (Pariante, 2017). GCR might therefore result in the resolution of a detectable association between cortisol and leukocyte differentials, which seems contradictory to the above mentioned assumption. Cole (2008), for instance, showed that the sensitivity of leukocytes to GCs was abrogated in the presence of a social stressor (loneliness). GCR was measured on the premise of a decrease or resolution of the relationship between cortisol levels and leukocyte counts. Despite the predictive value of HCC for the distribution of leukocyte differentials, Study 2 can be interpreted in line with the hypothesis of GCR, even if the study was not primarily designed to test for the stress-related abrogation of the association between HCC and leukocyte differentials. The basically positive correlational relationship between HCC and leukocyte differentials diminished or even disappeared under the influence of stress exposure due to the SLE, with restriction to neutrophils and lymphocytes. Interestingly, SLE did not show any effect on the relationship between the one-year change in HCC and monocytes (Figure 8). Considering that the change in HCC predicted the change in monocytes over one year, this association can be hypothesized as a pure physiological interaction between the

HPA axis and the immune system (Cain & Cidlowski, 2017; Webster et al., 2002). Similarly, Nikkheslat et al. (2015) compared patients suffering from CHD with and without depression. CHD patients with depression showed higher levels in all of the assessed inflammatory markers, whereas there was no difference in the number of monocytes between both groups. Why and how cortisol and monocytes can be associated at a physiological level but, independent of psychological stress exposure, remains to be an interesting research question for future exploration.

8.5   <u>Implementation of results in the stage model by Cohen and colleagues (2016)</u>

Results from Study 1 and Study 2 are in line with the stage model by Cohen et al. (2016), providing empirical evidence for the assumed levels (except 'poor health behavior'; stage model level 4, Figure 4). Summarized for a comprehensive interpretation, Study 1 and Study 2 support the hypothesis that chronic stress exposure must be appraised as stressful (level 2) and cause a negative emotional response (level 3) to affect subsequent levels. The fact that, in Study 2, the rating of how much an SLE affected a person the year prior to baseline assessment was associated with physiological alterations, whereas just the number of experienced events was not, supports the idea that level 2 and level 3 precede any further level. Environmental demands only (sum of SLE; level 1) could not predict a change in leukocyte differentials but demands measured by their appraisal (level 2) and emotional consequences (level 3). Alterations in the HPA axis activation with the result of changed cortisol levels interact with immune cells in such a way that the peripheral distribution of leukocytes is altered as well (level 5). With the only exception of monocytes, the interaction between cortisol and leukocyte differentials (neutrophils, lymphocytes) was not solely regulated on physiological level but was further influenced by environmental demands (SLE; level 1). Eventually, long-term changes in immune parameters (e.g. distribution of leukocytes) might open the gate to increased disease vulnerability (level 6), for instance, by the down-regulation of the overall immune defense. In line with Cohen et al. (2016), the results of this book support the significance of level 2 to level 5 to explain a potential pathway from chronic stress exposure to disease vulnerability and/or disease. The pathway that is suggested by this book is an altered HPA axis activation with the result of a changed availability of cortisol, which interacts with the distribution of leukocyte differentials. Due to increased neutrophils in the periphery and decreased lymphocytes, immune defense is hypothesized to be reduced in the long term and inflammatory processes increased (Figures 2 and 3). These processes are considered to open the gate to increased disease vulnerability and, lastly, to disease.

8.6 Extension of the stage model

8.6.1 Temporal dynamics in the adaptive stress response

Study 2 provides empirical support for the relevance of 'temporal dynamics' (level 7, Figure 4) as additional level within the stage model by Cohen et al. (2016). Temporal dynamics were assessed by a one-year change in the distribution of leukocyte differentials (level 5). The research model from Study 2 (Figure 7) proposed a continuous change in the distribution of leukocyte differentials, which was supported by the data for neutrophils and tentatively suggested for lymphocytes. Within the year between baseline assessment and follow-up, neutrophils showed an increase and lymphocytes a decrease in their peripheral distribution, due to the assessed stress exposure. Notably, the long-term distribution of leukocyte differentials was only based on two measurements, one at the baseline and the other at the follow-up one year later, without information about the time between both visits. Importantly, the conclusion of a continuous stress-related increase in neutrophils gained from Study 2 was assured by unpublished data from the second study follow-up.

Even if not explicitly tested in Study 1 or Study 2, temporal dynamics can be speculated as modulatory characteristic likewise acting on levels 1 to level 4. Temporal dynamics might, for instance, act on the experience of environmental demands (level 1) by the duration and timing of a stress exposure. With regard to stress exposure due to SLE, certain risk periods for the impact of adverse events on health-challenging effects can be considered. For example, effects of SLE on depression have been reported to be differential, dependent on the age at the time of occurrence (Kessler, 1997). Notably, not just the timing but also duration of the stress exposure is speculated to affect the adaptive stress response. For instance, stress exposure due to work overload needs to be sustained for at least six months for considering the burnout syndrome, which suggests that clinical relevance is associated with stress duration (Freedy & Hobfoll, 2017; Schaufeli et al., 2009; Van Der Klink & Van Dijk, 2003). It seems reasonable to speculate that the timing and duration of a stress exposure play an important role in the appraisal of the stressor (level 2) as well as for the emotional response (level 3). Only the lack of recovery from work stress as a function of time might lead to the appraisal that a stress exposure is challenging an individual's resources, resulting in a marked emotional response (Chrousos, 2009). Likewise, the timing and duration of a stress exposure are hypothesized to mediate the adaptive stress response at level of the HPA axis, as discussed in detail by Rohleder (2018; in regard to burnout) or Miller et al., (2007)

8.6.2 *Interactional dynamics: level 8*

Study 2 additionally assessed the temporal interaction between the HCC and the distribution of the leukocyte differentials, defined as 'interactional dynamics' (stage model by Cohen et al., 2016; level 8, Figure 4). Our data support the theory that stress-related changes in the HCC and in the distribution of leukocyte differentials (levels 4 and 5), cannot exclusively be explained by consideration of temporal dynamics within one physiological system, but by the long-term interaction between the HPA axis and the immune system. In addition, the interaction between altered leukocyte differentials (level 5) and poor health behavior (level 4) can be speculated for the following reason: Alterations in the distribution of leukocyte differentials coalesce with changed cytokine levels (Lotz et al., 1988; Ziegler-Heitbrock; 2007), with the consequence of a pathological surplus of pro- or anti-inflammatory cytokines (Figures 2 and 3). Cytokines communicate to the brain and can therefore influence behavioral, affective, and cognitive changes involved in the appraisal of sickness (Maier & Watkins, 1998). Cytokines might, for instance, participate in health-related behaviors such as the regulation of eating (review: Corcos et al., 2003) or sleeping behavior (systematic review: Irwin, Olmstead, & Carroll, 2015). In addition, the syndrome of cytokine-induced sickness behavior is defined by symptoms, such as weakness and listlessness, which combined form a motivational state to foster a certain behavioral output (Dantzer, 2004). Sickness behavior might be speculated to contribute to poor health behavior in the long term, for instance, by supporting lethargy/passivity, social withdrawal, and/or depressive mood.

8.6.3   *Completely developed disease: clinical implications*

'Completely developed disease' is considered the clinical endpoint of the stage model by Cohen et al. (2016, Figure 4). Neither the physiological paths assessed by Study 1 and Study 2, nor paths explored by theoretical research (Figures 1, 2, and 3) explain the stress-related progression of a specific disease outcome, but solely hypothesize a progression toward an overall increased vulnerability to adverse health conditions. Disease -related alterations (e.g. long-term up-/down-regulation of cortisol, continuous neutrophil increase) are speculated to cause increased disease vulnerability (level 6, figure 4). In line with the theory section (Chapters 2 and 3), a prolonged physiological stress response is defined as a risk factor for the switch from *allostasis* to *allostatic load/overload* (McEwen, 1998a, 1998b; McEwan & Wingfield, 2003), which emphasizes the importance of timing and duration as relevant characteristics in a potential pathway from stress exposure to disease (level 7). It seems reasonable to speculate that a final step from overall increased disease vulnerability (level 6) toward clinical manifestations of a certain mental or physical disease (level 9) may ensue from a slow process of physiological and behavioral alterations and likewise develop as a function of time (level 7).

8.6.4 *From chronic stress to disease: pathways supported by this book*

Empirical data from Study 1 and Study 2 can be embedded in the stage model by Cohen et al. (2016; Figure 4), as well as in the research model underlying this book (Figures 1, 2, and 3). Based on theoretical implications and empirical evidence, this book indicates potential pathways of how chronic stress exposure can contribute to every single level within the stage model, up to clinical manifestations of a certain disease. Apparently opposing conditions like, for example, those of hypercortisolemic, anti-inflammatory pathologies (Figure 2) as well as pathologies characterized by blunted HPA axis activity/GCR and a pro-inflammatory environment (Figure 3) are likewise explainable when considering time-dependent, dynamic alterations at the level of the HPA axis, for instance (Miller et al., 2007).

8.6.4.1 Thrombosis-associated and cardiovascular disease

Psychological stress is suggested to contribute to the development of pro-thrombotic states through alterations in blood flow and haemostasis (systematic review: Thrall, Lane, Carroll, & Lip, 2007). In line with a theory of protective immune response due to short-term stress exposure (Dhabhar, 2014), a pro-thrombotic state might protect the organism from excessive bleeding in case of injury in the context of a *fight-or-flight* response. A pro-thrombotic reaction may therefore be interpretable as an initially health- maintaining mechanism that turns health- challenging under the circumstances of chronic stress exposure (Austin et al., 2013). Stress-associated behaviors such as smoking, dieting, and/or alcohol consumption (level 4, figure 4) together with disease- related/HPA axis mediated (level 4) alterations such as increased blood pressure, pulse rate, and heart contractility (level 5), might contribute to increased vulnerability to thrombotic events (level 6; Hemingway & Marmot,

1999; Thrall et al., 2007). Study 2 suggests a continuous long-term alteration in the peripheral distribution of neutrophils due to chronic stress exposure. Considering that neutrophils amplify intravascular coagulation by forming neutrophil extracellular traps (Figure 2; Pfeiler et al., 2017), this book indicates evidence for a pathway from chronic stress exposure to thrombotic events. Given the contribution of neutrophils to the development of atherosclerosis (Gaul et al., 2017), a continuous stress-related increase in peripheral neutrophils might to some extent explain the association between stress exposure and CVD (Kivimäki & Kawachi, 2015; Steptoe & Kivimäki, 2013). Atherosclerosis is characterized by inflammation of the arterial vessel walls and can be assumed as clinical manifestation that precedes CVDs such as coronary heart disease (CHD) and strokes (Steptoe & Kivimäki, 2013). Interactions between neutrophils and platelets might further promote atherosclerosis and other inflammatory diseases (Brydon, Magid, & Steptoe, 2006; Zarbock, Polanowska-Grabowska, & Ley, 2007) and contribute to an increased disease vulnerability, which should be considered for future research projects.

8.7 Shortcomings and limitations

Study 1 and Study 2 were both assessed as part of the DBS and are both based on the same sample. Shortcomings due to study design and recruitment strategies are discussed in the study protocol (Penz, Wekenborg et al., 2018; Chapter 5). Indeed, when interpreting the results of this book, it needs to be considered that the conclusions are restricted to the specificity of the respective sample. The sample is lacking representative status for Germany or Dresden and shows a tendency toward strained individuals. The overestimation of strained individuals can be hypothesized to be due to the overriding aim of the DBS, namely the assessment of risk factors for burnout. Importantly, the assessment of chronic stress exposure as, it was operationalized in this book, is based on two distinct types of chronic stress exposure, namely burnout and cumulative SLE. In a narrow sense, the results from Study 1 and Study 2 should be interpreted solely on the basis of a certain stress experience and should not be mingled with a comprehensive conclusion. Certainly, both stressors share the characteristics of prolonged environmental demands which are appraised as stressful and trigger a negative emotional response (stage model by Cohen et al., 2016, level 1 to level 3, Figure 4), which serves as justification for an overall assumption. Several types of stressors should additionally be considered and validated in the future to generalize the extended stage model (Figure 4).

Even if this book aimed at theoretically and empirically addressing the issue of 'time' as an important determinant in the transmission from chronic stress exposure to increased disease vulnerability, our data do not provide the assessment of distinct physiological alterations throughout the life- span. Lupien, McEwen, Gunnar, and Heim (2009), for example, hypothesized that the physiological consequences of stress exposure vary at different stages of life. Different developmental stages of the brain regions such as the hippocampus or the amygdala, which participate in the regulation of the HPA axis activity, can be speculated to contribute differently to an adaptive stress response (review: Lupien et al., 2009).

Even though the results of this book support the hypothesis that physiological systems alter as a function of time, both studies assessed temporal dynamics in a rather narrow time window and restricted to a population of working age participants. In regard to Lupien et al. (2009), future studies should assess the influence of different developmental stages on the interaction between HPA axis activation and immune functions. There is already sound evidence that stress exposure during early developmental stages can trigger immunological pathologies in later life and that these pathologies in turn increase the vulnerability to cardiovascular, respiratory, metabolic, musculoskeletal, and autoimmune conditions (review: Miller, Chen, & Parker, 2011). It is an interesting research question for future projects to validate the results of this book on the basis of childhood stress exposure (e.g. childhood maltreatment, low socioeconomic status in childhood).

This book indicates a link between altered HPA axis activation/distribution of leukocyte differentials and inflammation/pro-inflammatory cytokines based on the fact that leukocytes secrete cytokines and can therefore participate in the promotion of a pro- inflammatory environment (Lotz et al., 1988; Smith, 1994). Neither Study 1 nor Study 2 assessed a direct measure of inflammation, such as IL-6 or CRP. In contrast to the assumption that the stress-related change in peripheral leukocytes promotes a health-challenging environment, monocytes – known to favor the production of pro-inflammatory cytokines (Ziegler-Heitbrock, 2007) – were not associated with chronic stress exposure in Study 2. Notably, in regard to this controversy, Figure 2 includes one paradox in its assumptions about the distribution of leukocyte differentials and inflammation: neutrophils are assumed to increase as a consequence of chronic stress exposure, which is supported by Study 2. Respectively Figure 2, the increase of neutrophils in the periphery is hypothesized to co-occur with an increase in the amount of available cortisol, which in turn is considered a promotor for an immuno-suppressive, anti-inflammatory environment. In contrast, neutrophils are suggested to induce a pro-inflammatory environment due to oxidative and enzymatic processes that foster tissue damage and inflammatory processes (Smith, 1994). Provided that every single path in Figure 2 and Figure 3 is correct, the paradox exemplifies that the physiological pathways which are involved in a long-term pathological stress response as described in the stage model by Cohen et al. (2016), develop in various complex interactions. Additionally, Figures 1 to 3 summarize single results, based on different samples and various kinds of stress exposure. It seems reasonable to speculate that many more pathological states might occur in relation to genetic and epigenetic predispositions, gender, age at stress experience, and dose-response effects, just to name a few.

Prospectively, validations of the current research model (Figures 1-4) should aim to include direct measures of inflammation and integrate these results into the extended stage model (Figure 4). For instance, it might be an interesting research question for future studies to combine measures of GCR (for instance, a single-dose overnight dexamethasone suppression test; Chrousos et al., 1993), assessment of pro- and anti-inflammatory cytokines, long/short-term measures of HPA axis activation (e.g. HCC and diurnal salivary cortisol), and the peripheral distribution of leukocyte differentials. The integration of these additional measures into an overall model that combines the stage model by Cohen et al. (2016) plus the suggested extensions of the stage model, and the interaction pathways described in Figures 1, 2, and 3 will provide profound and detailed understanding of the mechanisms that constitute that pathway between chronic stress exposure and disease. Additionally, a validation and/or exploration of the clinical relevance of the respective stress-related physiological alterations is suggested. For instance, the results of this book provide evidence for a long-term increase in neutrophils months or even years after stress cessation. It needs to be clarified in future multi-disciplinary projects whether, or when, statistically significant physiological alterations turn into a health-threatening condition.

9 Conclusion

Despite the above discussed limitations, this book shows potential pathways of how chronic stress exposure can enter and *stay in* the body for a long time after stress cessation. Our results provide evidence for a long-term alteration at the level of the HPA axis which is suggested to up-regulate the availability of cortisol in response to a chronic stressor (burnout). Furthermore, chronic stress exposure is suggested to contribute to long-term alterations in the peripheral distribution of leukocyte differentials, specified for neutrophils. The long-term interactional dynamics shown for cortisol and leukocyte differentials attenuated or diminished due to the experience of stressful life events, which supports the theory of GCR.

Considering that the number and proportion of leukocyte differentials in the blood represents the state of activation of the immune system and its defense mechanisms, this book suggests a direct pathway between stress exposure and increased vulnerability to adverse health conditions. An adaptive HPA axis and immunologic stress response, as it is suggested by this book, provides an explanation for the association between chronic stress exposure and clinical manifestation, such as inflammatory and/or autoimmune diseases shown in several cross-sectional studies. Considering the temporal and interactional dynamics of the respective physiological systems, apparently controversial clinical manifestations, such as immuno-suppressive/anti-inflammatory as well as immuno-active/pro-inflammatory environments, are likewise explainable.

10 References

Afari, N., & Buchwald, D. (2014). Chronic fatigue syndrome: a review. *American Journal of Psychiatry, 160*, 221-236.

Ahola, K., Honkonen, T., Isometsä, E., Kalimo, R., Nykyri, E., Aromaa, A., & Lönnqvist, J. (2005). The relationship between job-related burnout and depressive disorders - results from the Finnish Health 2000 Study. *Journal of affective disorders, 88*, 55-62.

Ahola, K., Väänänen, A., Koskinen, A., Kouvonen, A., & Shirom, A. (2010). Burnout as a predictor of all-cause mortality among industrial employees: a 10-year prospective register-linkage study. *Journal of psychosomatic research, 69*, 51-57.

Andel, R., Crowe, M., Hahn, E. A., Mortimer, J. A., Pedersen, N. L., Fratiglioni, L., . . . Gatz, M. (2012). Work-related stress may increase the risk of vascular dementia. *Journal of the American Geriatrics Society, 60*, 60-67.

Alarcon, G., Eschleman, K. J., & Bowling, N. A. (2009). Relationships between personality variables and burnout: A meta-analysis. *Work & Stress, 23*, 244-263.

American Psychiatric Association (2013). Diagnostic and statistical manual of mental disorders (DSM-5®): American Psychiatric Pub.

Auffray, C., Sieweke, M. H., & Geissmann, F. (2009). Blood monocytes: development, heterogeneity, and relationship with dendritic cells. *Annual review of immunology, 27*, 669-692.

Austin, A. W., Wissmann, T., & von Känel, R. (2013). Stress and hemostasis: an update. *Seminars in thrombosis and hemostasis, 39*, 902-912.

Avitsur, R., Stark, J. L., & Sheridan, J. F. (2001). Social stress induces glucocorticoid resistance in subordinate animals. *Hormones and Behavior, 39*, 247-257.

Backhaus, J., Junghanns, K., Broocks, A., Riemann, D., & Hohagen, F. (2002). Test–retest reliability and validity of the Pittsburgh Sleep Quality Index in primary insomnia. *Journal of Psychosomatic Research, 53*, 737-740.

Backhaus, J., Junghanns, K., & Hohagen, F. (2004). Sleep disturbances are correlated with decreased morning awakening salivary cortisol. *Psychoneuroendocrinology, 29*, 1184-1191.

Bakusic, J., Schaufeli, W., Claes, S., and Godderis, L. (2017). Stress , burnout and depression : A systematic review on DNA methylation mechanisms. *Journal of Psychosomatic Research, 92*, 34–44.

Barnes, P. J. (2010). Mechanisms and resistance in glucocorticoid control of inflammation. *The Journal of steroid biochemistry and molecular biology, 120*, 76-85.

Barnes, P. J., & Adcock, I. M. (2009). Glucocorticoid resistance in inflammatory diseases. *The Lancet, 373*, 1905-1917.

Baumeister, D., Akhtar, R., Ciufolini, S., Pariante, C., & Mondelli, V. (2015). Childhood trauma and adulthood inflammation: a meta-analysis of peripheral C-reactive protein, interleukin-6 and tumour necrosis factor-α. *Molecular psychiatry, 21*, 642-649.

Baumeister, D., Lightman, S. L., & Pariante, C. M. (2016). The HPA Axis in the Pathogenesis and Treatment of Depressive Disorders: Integrating Clinical and Molecular Findings. *Psychopathology Review, 3*, 64-76.

Baumeister, D., Russell, A., Pariante, C. M., & Mondelli, V. (2014). Inflammatory biomarker profiles of mental disorders and their relation to clinical, social and lifestyle factors. *Social psychiatry and psychiatric epidemiology, 49*, 841-849.

Beards, S., Gayer-Anderson, C., Borges, S., Dewey, M. E., Fisher, H. L., & Morgan, C. (2013). Life events and psychosis: a review and meta-analysis. *Schizophrenia bulletin, 39*, 740-747.

Benjet, C., Bromet, E., Karam, E., Kessler, R., McLaughlin, K., Ruscio, A., . . . Hill, E. (2016). The epidemiology of traumatic event exposure worldwide: results from the World Mental Health Survey Consortium. *Psychological medicine, 46*, 327-343.

Beser, A., Sorjonen, K., Wahlberg, K., Peterson, U., Nygren, A., & Asberg, M. (2014). Construction and evaluation of a self rating scale for stress-induced Exhaustion Disorder, the Karolinska Exhaustion Disorder Scale. *Scandinavian journal of psychology, 55*, 72-82.

Bianchi, R., Boffy, C., Hingray, C., Truchot, D., & Laurent, E. (2013). Comparative symptomatology of burnout and depression. *Journal of health psychology, 18*, 782-787.

Bianchi, R., Schonfeld, I. S., & Laurent, E. (2015). Burnout-depression overlap: A review. *Clinical Psychology Review, 36*, 28-41.

Bless, H., Wanke, M., Bohner, G., Fellhauer, R., & Schwarz, N. (1994). Need for cognition- a scale measuring engagement and hapiness in cognitive tasks. *Zeitschrift für Sozialpsychologie, 25*, 147-154

Blom, V., Bergström, G., Hallsten, L., Bodin, L., and Svedberg, P. (2012). Genetic susceptibility to burnout in a Swedish twin cohort. *European Journal of Epidemiology, 27*, 225–231.

Booij, S. H., Bouma, E. M., de Jonge, P., Ormel, J., & Oldehinkel, A. J. (2013). Chronicity of depressive problems and the cortisol response to psychosocial stress in adolescents: The TRAILS study. *Psychoneuroendocrinology, 38*, 659-666.

Borritz, M., Christensen, K. B., Bültmann, U., Rugulies, R., Lund, T., Andersen, I., . . . Kristensen, T. S. (2010). Impact of burnout and psychosocial work characteristics on future long-term sickness absence. Prospective results of the Danish PUMA Study among human service workers. *Journal of Occupational and Environmental Medicine, 52*, 964-970.

Brydon, L., Magid, K., & Steptoe, A. (2006). Platelets, coronary heart disease, and stress. *Brain, behavior, and immunity, 20*, 113-119.

Bullinger, M., Kirchberger, I., & Ware, J. (1995). Der deutsche SF-36 Health Survey. Übersetzung und psychometrische Testung eines krankheitsübergreifenden Instruments zur Erfassung der gesundheitsbezogenen Lebensqualität. *Zeitschrift für Gesundheitswissenschaften=Journal of public health, 3*, 21-36.

Bundespsychotherapeutenkammer, BPtK. (2012). Studie zur Arbeitsunfähigkeit, psychische Erkrankungen und Burnout.

Büssing, A., & Glaser, J. (1999). Deutsche Fassung des Maslach Burnout Inventory–General Survey (MBI-GS-D). *München, Technische Universität, Lehrstuhl für Psychologie.*

Cain, D. W., & Cidlowski, J. A. (2017). Immune regulation by glucocorticoids. *Nature Reviews Immunology, 17*, 233-247.

Cattaneo, A., Macchi, F., Plazzotta, G., Veronica, B., Bocchio-Chiavetto, L., Riva, M. A., & Pariante, C. M. (2015). Inflammation and neuronal plasticity: a link between childhood trauma and depression pathogenesis. *Frontiers in cellular neuroscience, 9*, 1-12.

Chida, Y., & Steptoe, A. (2009). The association of anger and hostility with future coronary heart disease: a meta-analytic review of prospective evidence. *Journal of the American college of cardiology, 53*, 936-946.

Choi, K. R., Kim, D., Jang, E. Y., Bae, H., & Kim, S. H. (2017). Reliability and Validity of the Korean Version of the Lifetime Stressor Checklist-Revised in Psychiatric Outpatients with Anxiety or Depressive Disorders. *Yonsei medical journal, 58*, 226-233.

Christensen, H., & Boysen, G. (2004). C-reactive protein and white blood cell count increases in the first 24 hours after acute stroke. *Cerebrovascular diseases, 18*, 214-219.

Chrousos, G. P. (2009). Stress and disorders of the stress system. *Nature Reviews Endocrinology, 5*, 374-381.

Chrousos, G. P., Detera-Wadleigh, S. D., & Karl, M. (1993). Syndromes of glucocorticoid resistance. *Annals of Internal Medicine, 119*, 1113-1124.

Cleare, A. J. (2004). The HPA axis and the genesis of chronic fatigue syndrome. *Trends in Endocrinology & Metabolism, 15*, 55-59.

Coelho, R., Viola, T., Walss-Bass, C., Brietzke, E., & Grassi-Oliveira, R. (2014). Childhood maltreatment and inflammatory markers: a systematic review. *Acta Psychiatrica Scandinavica, 129*, 180-192.

Cohen, S., Gianaros, P. J., & Manuck, S. B. (2016). A stage model of stress and disease. *Perspectives on Psychological Science, 11*, 456-463.

Cohen, S., Janicki-Deverts, D., Doyle, W. J., Miller, G. E., Frank, E., Rabin, B. S., & Turner, R. B. (2012). Chronic stress, glucocorticoid receptor resistance, inflammation, and disease risk. *Proceedings of the National Academy of Sciences, 109*, 5995-5999.

Cohen, S., Janicki-Deverts, D., & Miller, G. E. (2007). Psychological stress and disease. *Jama, 298*, 1685-1687.

Cohen, S., Kessler, R. C., & Gordon, L. U. (1995). Strategies for measuring stress in studies of psychiatric and physical disorders. *Measuring stress: A guide for health and social scientists*. Oxford University Press, 3-26.

Cole, S. W. (2008). Social regulation of leukocyte homeostasis: the role of glucocorticoid sensitivity. *Brain, behavior, and immunity, 22*, 1049-1055.

Corcos, M., Guilbaud, O., Paterniti, S., Moussa, M., Chambry, J., Chaouat, G., . . . Jeammet, P. (2003). Involvement of cytokines in eating disorders: a critical review of the human literature. *Psychoneuroendocrinology, 28*, 229-249.

Danese, A., Moffitt, T. E., Pariante, C. M., Ambler, A., Poulton, R., & Caspi, A. (2008). Elevated inflammation levels in depressed adults with a history of childhood maltreatment. *Archives of general psychiatry, 65*, 409-415.

Danese, A., Pariante, C. M., Caspi, A., Taylor, A., & Poulton, R. (2007). Childhood maltreatment predicts adult inflammation in a life-course study. *Proceedings of the National Academy of Sciences, 104*, 1319-1324.

Danhof-Pont, M. B., van Veen, T., & Zitman, F. G. (2011). Biomarkers in burnout: a systematic review. *Journal of psychosomatic research, 70*, 505-524.

Dantzer, R. (2004). Cytokine-induced sickness behaviour: a neuroimmune response to activation of innate immunity. *European journal of pharmacology, 500*, 399-411.

Dantzer, R. (2009). Cytokine, sickness behavior, and depression. *Immunology and Allergy Clinics, 29*, 247-264.

De Kloet, E. R., Joëls, M., & Holsboer, F. (2005). Stress and the brain: from adaptation to disease. *Nature Reviews Neuroscience, 6*, 463-475.

De Vente, W., van Amsterdam, J. G., Olff, M., Kamphuis, J. H., & Emmelkamp, P. M. (2015). Burnout is associated with reduced parasympathetic activity and reduced HPA axis responsiveness, predominantly in males. *BioMed research international, 2015*, article ID 431725.

Deinzer, R., Kirschbaum, C., Gresele, C., & Hellhammer, D. (1997). Adrenocortical responses to repeated parachute jumping and subsequent h-CRH challenge in inexperienced healthy subjects. *Physiology & behavior, 61*, 507-511.

Deligkaris, P., Panagopoulou, E., Montgomery, A. J., & Masoura, E. (2014). Job burnout and cognitive functioning: A systematic review. *Work & Stress, 28*, 107-123.

Delves, P. J., & Roitt, I. M. (2000). The immune system. *New England journal of medicine, 343*, 37-49.

Demitrack, M. A., Dale, J. K., Straus, S. E., Laue, L., Listwak, S. J., Kruesi, M. J., . . . Gold, P. W. (1991). Evidence for impaired activation of the hypothalamic-pituitary-adrenal axis in patients with chronic fatigue syndrome. *The Journal of Clinical Endocrinology & Metabolism, 73*, 1224-1234.

Dettenborn, L., Muhtz, C., Skoluda, N., Stalder, T., Steudte, S., Hinkelmann, K., . . . Otte, C. (2012). Introducing a novel method to assess cumulative steroid concentrations: increased hair cortisol concentrations over 6 months in medicated patients with depression. *Stress, 15*, 348-353.

Dhabhar, F. S. (2002). Stress-induced augmentation of immune function—the role of stress hormones, leukocyte trafficking, and cytokines. *Brain, behavior, and immunity, 16*, 785-798.

Dhabhar, F. S. (2014). Effects of stress on immune function: the good, the bad, and the beautiful. *Immunologic Research, 58*, 193-210.

Dhabhar, F. S., Malarkey, W. B., Neri, E., & McEwen, B. S. (2012). Stress-induced redistribution of immune cells—From barracks to boulevards to battlefields: A tale of three hormones–Curt Richter Award Winner. *Psychoneuroendocrinology, 37*, 1345-1368.

Dhabhar, F. S., & Mcewen, B. S. (1997). Acute stress enhances while chronic stress suppresses cell-mediated immunity in vivo: A potential role for leukocyte trafficking. *Brain, behavior, and immunity, 11*, 286-306.

Dickerson, S. S., & Kemeny, M. E. (2004). Acute stressors and cortisol responses: a theoretical integration and synthesis of laboratory research. *Psychological bulletin, 130*, 355-391.

Dimsdale, J. E. (2008). Psychological stress and cardiovascular disease. *Journal of the American college of cardiology, 51*, 1237-1246.

Dormann, C., & Griffin, M. A. (2015). Optimal time lags in panel studies. *Psychological Methods, 20*, 489-505.

Ehlert, U., Gaab, J., & Heinrichs, M. (2001). Psychoneuroendocrinological contributions to the etiology of depression, posttraumatic stress disorder, and stress-related bodily disorders: the role of the hypothalamus–pituitary–adrenal axis. *Biological psychology, 57*, 141-152.

Elenkov, I. J. (2004). Glucocorticoids and the Th1/Th2 balance. *Annals of the New York Academy of Sciences, 1024*, 138-146.

Elenkov, I. J., & Chrousos, G. P. (1999). Stress hormones, Th1/Th2 patterns, pro/anti-inflammatory cytokines and susceptibility to disease. *Trends in Endocrinology & Metabolism, 10*, 359-368.

Elenkov, I. J., & Chrousos, G. P. (2006). Stress system–organization, physiology and immunoregulation. *Neuroimmunomodulation, 13*, 257-267.

Engler, H., Bailey, M. T., Engler, A., & Sheridan, J. F. (2004). Effects of repeated social stress on leukocyte distribution in bone marrow, peripheral blood and spleen. *Journal of neuroimmunology, 148*, 106-115.

Evolahti, A., Hultell, D., & Collins, A. (2013). Development of burnout in middle-aged working women: A longitudinal study. *Journal of women's health, 22*, 94-103.

Foster, R. G., & Roenneberg, T. (2008). Human responses to the geophysical daily, annual and lunar cycles. *Current Biology, 18*, R784-R794.

Fliege, H., Rose, M., Arck, P., Levenstein, S., & Klapp, B. (2001). Validierung des " Perceived Stress Questionnaire"(PSQ) an einer deutschen Stichprobe. *Diagnostica, 47*, 142-152.

Franchimont, D., Kino, T., Galon, J., Meduri, G. U., & Chrousos, G. (2002). Glucocorticoids and inflammation revisited: the state of the art. *Neuroimmunomodulation, 10*, 247-260.

Freedy, J., & Hobfoll, S. E. (2017). Conservation of resources: A general stress theory applied to burnout. *Professional burnout* (pp. 115-129): Routledge.

Friedl, P., & Weigelin, B. (2008). Interstitial leukocyte migration and immune function. *Nature immunology, 9*, 960-969.

Fries, E., Hesse, J., Hellhammer, J., & Hellhammer, D. H. (2005). A new view on hypocortisolism. *Psychoneuroendocrinology, 30*, 1010-1016.

Gao, W., Stalder, T., Foley, P., Rauh, M., Deng, H., & Kirschbaum, C. (2013). Quantitative analysis of steroid hormones in human hair using a column-switching LC–APCI–MS/MS assay. *Journal of Chromatography B, 928*, 1-8.

Gao, W., Kirschbaum, C., Grass, J., & Stalder, T. (2016). LC–MS based analysis of endogenous steroid hormones in human hair. *The Journal of Steroid Biochemistry and Molecular Biology, 162*, 92-99.

Garnefski, N., Kraaij, V., & Spinhoven, P. (2001). Negative life events, cognitive emotion regulation and emotional problems. *Personality and Individual Differences, 30*, 1311-1327.

Gaul, D. S., Stein, S., & Matter, C. M. (2017). Neutrophils in cardiovascular disease. *European Heart Journal, 38*, 1702-1704.

Gerber, M., Kalak, N., Elliot, C., Holsboer-Trachsler, E., Pühse, U., & Brand, S. (2013). Both hair cortisol levels and perceived stress predict increased symptoms of depression: an exploratory study in young adults. *Neuropsychobiology, 68*, 100-109.

Geurts, S. A., Taris, T. W., Kompier, M. A., Dikkers, J. S., Van Hooff, M. L., & Kinnunen, U. M. (2005). Work-home interaction from a work psychological perspective: Development and validation of a new questionnaire, the SWING. *Work & Stress, 19*, 319-339.

Gillies, J., & Neimeyer, R. A. (2006). Loss, grief, and the search for significance: Toward a model of meaning reconstruction in bereavement. *Journal of Constructivist Psychology, 19*, 31-65.

Glaser, R., & Kiecolt-Glaser, J. K. (2005). Stress-induced immune dysfunction: implications for health. *Nature Reviews Immunology, 5*, 243-251.

Glaser, R., Kiecolt-Glaser, J. K., Marucha, P. T., MacCallum, R. C., Laskowski, B. F., & Malarkey, W. B. (1999). Stress-related changes in proinflammatory cytokine production in wounds. *Archives of general psychiatry, 56*, 450-456.

Golbidi, S., Frisbee, J. C., & Laher, I. (2015). Chronic stress impacts the cardiovascular system: animal models and clinical outcomes. *American Journal of Physiology-Heart and Circulatory Physiology, 308*, H1476-H1498.

Grass, J., Miller, R., Carlitz, E. H., Patrovsky, F., Gao, W., Kirschbaum, C., & Stalder, T. (2016). In vitro influence of light radiation on hair steroid concentrations. *Psychoneuroendocrinology, 73*, 109-116.

Grossi, G., Perski, A., Osika, W., & Savic, I. (2015). Stress-related exhaustion disorder–clinical manifestation of burnout? A review of assessment methods, sleep impairments, cognitive disturbances, and neuro-biological and physiological changes in clinical burnout. *Scandinavian journal of psychology, 56*, 626-636.

Grossi, G., Perski, A., Evengård, B., Blomkvist, V., & Orth-Gomér, K. (2003). Physiological correlates of burnout among women. *Journal of Psychosomatic Research, 55*, 309–316.

Grossi, G., Theorell, T., Jürisoo, M., and Setterlind, S. (1999). Psychophysiological correlates of organizational change and threat of unemployment among police inspectors. *Integrative Physiological and Behavioral Science, 34*, 30–42.

Hakanen, J. J., & Schaufeli, W. B. (2012). Do burnout and work engagement predict depressive symptoms and life satisfaction? A three-wave seven-year prospective study. *Journal of affective disorders, 141*, 415-424.

Halbesleben, J. R., & Demerouti, E. (2005). The construct validity of an alternative measure of burnout: Investigating the English translation of the Oldenburg Burnout Inventory. *Work & Stress, 19*, 208-220.

Hänsel, A., Hong, S., Cámara, R. J., & Von Kaenel, R. (2010). Inflammation as a psychophysiological biomarker in chronic psychosocial stress. *Neuroscience & Biobehavioral Reviews, 35*, 115-121.

Hathaway, L. M., Boals, A., & Banks, J. B. (2010). PTSD symptoms and dominant emotional response to a traumatic event: an examination of DSM-IV Criterion A2. *Anxiety, Stress & Coping, 23*, 119-126.

Heim, C., Ehlert, U., & Hellhammer, D. H. (2000). The potential role of hypocortisolism in the pathophysiology of stress-related bodily disorders. *Psychoneuroendocrinology, 25*, 1-35.

Heim, C., Nater, U. M., Maloney, E., Boneva, R., Jones, J. F., & Reeves, W. C. (2009). Childhood trauma and risk for chronic fatigue syndrome: association with neuroendocrine dysfunction. *Archives of general psychiatry, 66*, 72-80.

Hemingway, H., & Marmot, M. (1999). Psychosocial factors in the aetiology and prognosis of coronary heart disease: systematic review of prospective cohort studies. *Bmj, 318*, 1460-1467.

Henley, D., & Lightman, S. (2011). New insights into corticosteroid-binding globulin and glucocorticoid delivery. *Neuroscience, 180*, 1-8.

Herane-Vives, A., Angel, V., Papadopoulos, A., Wise, T., Chua, K. C., Strawbridge, R., . . . Cleare, A. (2018). Short-term and long-term measures of cortisol in saliva and hair in atypical and non-atypical depression. *Acta Psychiatrica Scandinavica, 137*, 216-230.

Herr, R. M., Almer, C., Loerbroks, A., Barrech, A., Elfantel, I., Siegrist, J., . . . Li, J. (2018). Associations of work stress with hair cortisol concentrations–initial findings from a prospective study. *Psychoneuroendocrinology, 89*, 134-137.

Hinkelmann, K., Muhtz, C., Dettenborn, L., Agorastos, A., Wingenfeld, K., Spitzer, C., . . . Otte, C. (2013). Association between childhood trauma and low hair cortisol in depressed patients and healthy control subjects. *Biological psychiatry, 74*, e15-e17.

Horne, B. D., Anderson, J. L., John, J. M., Weaver, A., Bair, T. L., Jensen, K. R., . . . Muhlestein, J. B. (2005). Which white blood cell subtypes predict increased cardiovascular risk? *Journal of the American college of cardiology, 45*, 1638-1643.

Huibers, M., Beurskens, A., Prins, J., Kant, I., Bazelmans, E., Van Schayck, C., . . . Bleijenberg, G. (2003). Fatigue, burnout, and chronic fatigue syndrome among employees on sick leave: do attributions make the difference? *Occupational and environmental medicine, 60*, i26-i31.

Humphreys, J. C., Bernal De Pheils, P., Slaughter, R. E., Uribe, T., Jaramillo, D., Tiwari, A., . . . Belknap, R. A. (2011). Translation and adaptation of the life stressor checklist-revised with Colombian women. *Health care for women international, 32*, 599-612.

Hunter, C. A., & Jones, S. A. (2015). IL-6 as a keystone cytokine in health and disease. *Nature immunology, 16*, 448-457.

Irwin, M. R., Olmstead, R., & Carroll, J. E. (2015). Sleep disturbance, sleep duration, and inflammation: a systematic review and meta-analysis of cohort studies and experimental sleep deprivation. *Biological psychiatry, 80*, 40-52.

Janssens, H., Clays, E., Fiers, T., Verstraete, A., De Bacquer, D., & Braeckman, L. (2017). Hair cortisol in relation to job stress and depressive symptoms. *Occupational Medicine, 67*, 114-120.

Jarczok, M. N., Jarczok, M., Mauss, D., Koenig, J., Li, J., Herr, R. M., & Thayer, J. F. (2013). Autonomic nervous system activity and workplace stressors—A systematic review. *Neuroscience & Biobehavioral Reviews, 37*, 1810-1823.

John, O. P., Donahue, E. M., & Kentle, R. L. (1991). The big five inventory—versions 4a and 54. Berkeley, CA: University of California, Berkeley, Institute of Personality and Social Research.

Jönsson, P., Österberg, K., Wallergård, M., Hansen, Å. M., Garde, A. H., Johansson, G., & Karlson, B. (2015). Exhaustion-related changes in cardiovascular and cortisol reactivity to acute psychosocial stress. *Physiology & behavior, 151*, 327-337.

Juruena, M. F., Bocharova, M., Agustini, B., & Young, A. H. (2018). Atypical depression and non-atypical depression: Is HPA axis function a biomarker? A systematic review. *Journal of affective disorders, 233*, 45-67.

Juster, R.-P., Sindi, S., Marin, M.-F., Perna, A., Hashemi, A., Pruessner, J. C., & Lupien, S. J. (2011). A clinical allostatic load index is associated with burnout symptoms and hypocortisolemic profiles in healthy workers. *Psychoneuroendocrinology, 36*, 797-805.

Kalimo, R., Pahkin, K., Mutanen, P., & Topipinen-Tanner, S. (2003). Staying well or burning out at work: work characteristics and personal resources as long-term predictors. *Work & Stress, 17*, 109-122.

Kanthak, M. K., Stalder, T., Hill, L., Thayer, J. F., Penz, M., & Kirschbaum, C. (2017). Autonomic dysregulation in burnout and depression: evidence for the central role of exhaustion. *Scandinavian Journal of Work, Environment & Health, 43*, 475 - 484.

Kaplanski, G., Marin, V., Montero-Julian, F., Mantovani, A., & Farnarier, C. (2003). IL-6: a regulator of the transition from neutrophil to monocyte recruitment during inflammation. *Trends in immunology, 24*, 25-29.

Kaschka, W. P., Korczak, D., & Broich, K. (2011). Burnout: A fashionable diagnosis. *Deutsches Ärzteblatt International, 108*, 781-787.

Kendler, K. S., Karkowski, L. M., & Prescott, C. A. (1999). Causal relationship between stressful life events and the onset of major depression. *American Journal of Psychiatry, 156*, 837-841.

Kessler, R. C. (1997). The effects of stressful life events on depression. *Annual review of psychology, 48*, 191-214.

Keyes, K. M., McLaughlin, K. A., Demmer, R. T., Cerdá, M., Koenen, K. C., Uddin, M., & Galea, S. (2013). Potentially traumatic events and the risk of six physical health conditions in a population-based sample. *Depression and anxiety, 30*, 451-460.

Kiecolt-Glaser, J. K., Marucha, P. T., Mercado, A., Malarkey, W. B., & Glaser, R. (1995). Slowing of wound healing by psychological stress. *The Lancet, 346*, 1194-1196.

Kilpeläinen, M., Koskenvuo, M., Helenius, H., & Terho, E. (2002). Stressful life events promote the manifestation of asthma and atopic diseases. *Clinical & Experimental Allergy, 32*, 256-263.

Kirschbaum, C., Pirke, K.-M., & Hellhammer, D. H. (1993). The 'Trier Social Stress Test'–a tool for investigating psychobiological stress responses in a laboratory setting. *Neuropsychobiology, 28*, 76-81.

Kirschbaum, C., Tietze, A., Skoluda, N., & Dettenborn, L. (2009). Hair as a retrospective calendar of cortisol production—increased cortisol incorporation into hair in the third trimester of pregnancy. *Psychoneuroendocrinology, 34*, 32-37.

Kivimäki, M., & Kawachi, I. (2015). Work stress as a risk factor for cardiovascular disease. *Current cardiology reports, 17*, 74.

Kleijweg J. H. M, Verbraak M. J. P. M., Van Dijk M. K. (2013). The clinical utility of the Maslach Burnout Inventory in a clinical population. Psychol Assess 25, 435–441.

Kocalevent, R. D., Klapp, B. F., Albani, C., & Brähler, E. (2013). Zusammenhänge von Ressourcen, chronisch aktiviertem Distress und Erschöpfung in der deutschen Allgemeinbevölkerung. *Psychotherapie Psychosomatik Medizinische Psychologie, 63*, 115-121.

Korczak, D., Huber, B., & Kister, C. (2010). Differential diagnostic of the burnout syndrome. *GMS health technology assessment, 6,* ISSN 1861-8863.

Korczak, D., Kister, C., & Huber, B. (2008). *Differentialdiagnostik des Burnout-Syndroms.* DIMDI, Köln 2010.

Kovaleva, A., Beierlein, C., Kemper, C., & Rammstedt, B. (2012). Eine Kurzskala zur Messung von Kontrollüberzeugung: *Die Skala Internale-Externale-Kontrollüberzeugung-4 (IE-4).* Mannheim: GESIS-Leipniz Institut für Sozialwissenschaften. Retrieved: http://nbn-resolving.de/urn:nbn:de:0168-ssoar-312096

Kraan, T., Velthorst, E., Smit, F., de Haan, L., & van der Gaag, M. (2015). Trauma and recent life events in individuals at ultra high risk for psychosis: review and meta-analysis. *Schizophrenia research, 161,* 143-149.

Kratofil, R. M., Kubes, P., & Deniset, J. F. (2017). Monocyte conversion during inflammation and injury. *Arteriosclerosis, thrombosis, and vascular biology, 37,* 35-42.

Kristensen, T. S., Borritz, M., Villadsen, E., & Christensen, K. B. (2005). The Copenhagen Burnout Inventory: A new tool for the assessment of burnout. *Work & Stress, 19,* 192-207.

Kroenke, K., Spitzer, R. L., & Williams, J. B. (2001). The Phq-9. *Journal of general internal medicine, 16,* 606-613.

Kudielka, B. M., Hellhammer, D., & Wüst, S. (2009). Why do we respond so differently? Reviewing determinants of human salivary cortisol responses to challenge. *Psychoneuroendocrinology, 34,* 2-18.

Kudielka, B. M., Schommer, N. C., Hellhammer, D. H., & Kirschbaum, C. (2004). Acute HPA axis responses, heart rate, and mood changes to psychosocial stress (TSST) in humans at different times of day. *Psychoneuroendocrinology, 29,* 983-992.

Kudielka B. M., & Wüst, S. (2010). Human models in acute and chronic stress: assessing determinants of individual hypothalamus–pituitary–adrenal axis activity and reactivity. *Stress, 13,* 1-14.

Lagraauw, H. M., Kuiper, J., & Bot, I. (2015). Acute and chronic psychological stress as risk factors for cardiovascular disease: Insights gained from epidemiological, clinical and experimental studies. *Brain, behavior, and immunity, 50,* 18-30.

Lavoie, J. A., & Douglas, K. S. (2012). The Perceived Stress Scale: Evaluating configural, metric and scalar invariance across mental health status and gender. *Journal of Psychopathology and Behavioral Assessment, 34,* 48-57.

Leiter, M. P., Hakanen, J. J., Ahola, K., Toppinen-Tanner, S., Koskinen, A., & Väänänen, A. (2013). Organizational predictors and health consequences of changes in burnout: A 12-year cohort study. *Journal of Organizational Behavior, 34,* 959-973.

Leka, S., Jain, A. (2010). *Health impact of psychosocial hazards at work: an overview.* Geneva: World Helath Organisation. Retrieved from http://apps.who.int/iris/bitstream/10665/44428/1/9789241500272_eng.pdf

Lennartsson, A.-K., Billig, H., & Jonsdottir, I. H. (2014). Burnout is associated with elevated prolactin levels in men but not in women. *Journal of Psychosomatic Research, 76,* 380–383.

Leone, S. S., Wessely, S., Huibers, M. J., Knottnerus, J. A., & Kant, I. (2011). Two sides of the same coin? On the history and phenomenology of chronic fatigue and burnout. *Psychology and Health, 26,* 449-464.

Levenstein, S., Prantera, C., Varvo, V., Scribano, M. L., Berto, E., Luzi, C., & Andreoli, A. (1993). Development of the Perceived Stress Questionnaire: a new tool for psychosomatic research. *Journal of Psychosomatic Research, 37,* 19-32.

Lindwall, M., Gerber, M., Jonsdottir, I. H., Börjesson, M., & Ahlborg Jr, G. (2014). The relationships of change in physical activity with change in depression, anxiety, and burnout: A longitudinal study of Swedish healthcare workers. *Health Psychology, 33*, 1309-1318.

Lock, S., Rubin, G. J., Murray, V., Rogers, M. B., Amlôt, R., & Williams, R. (2012). Secondary stressors and extreme events and disasters: a systematic review of primary research from 2010-2011. *PLoS currents, 29, 4.*

Lotz, M., Vaughan, J. H., & Carson, D. A. (1988). Effect of neuropeptides on production of inflammatory cytokines by human monocytes. *Science, 241*, 1218-1222.

Löwe, B., Decker, O., Müller, S., Brähler, E., Schellberg, D., Herzog, W., & Herzberg, P. Y. (2008). Validation and standardization of the Generalized Anxiety Disorder Screener (GAD-7) in the general population. *Medical Care, 46*, 266-274.

Löwe, B., Spitzer, R., Zipfel, S., & Herzog, W. (2002). PHQ-D. *Gesundheitsfragebogen für Patienten*, 2. Auflage. Karlsruhe: Pfitzer.

Lupien, S. J., McEwen, B. S., Gunnar, M. R., & Heim, C. (2009). Effects of stress throughout the lifespan on the brain, behaviour and cognition. *Nature Reviews Neuroscience, 10*, 434-445.

MacCallum, R., Zhang, S., Preacher, K. J., & Rucker, D. D. (2002). On the practice of dichotomization of qualitative variables. *Psychological Methods, 7*, 19-40.

Maier, S. F., & Watkins, L. R. (1998). Cytokines for psychologists: implications of bidirectional immune-to-brain communication for understanding behavior, mood, and cognition. *Psychological review, 105*, 83-107.

Malarkey, W. B., Pearl, D. K., Demers, L. M., Kiecolt-Glaser, J. K., & Glaser, R. (1995). Influence of academic stress and season on 24-hour mean concentrations of ACTH, cortisol, and β-endorphin. *Psychoneuroendocrinology, 20*, 499-508.

Manenschijn, L., Schaap, L., Van Schoor, N., van der Pas, S., Peeters, G., Lips, P., . . . Van Rossum, E. (2013). High long-term cortisol levels, measured in scalp hair, are associated with a history of cardiovascular disease. *The Journal of Clinical Endocrinology & Metabolism, 98*, 2078-2083.

Marchand, A., Juster, R.-P., Durand, P., & Lupien, S. J. (2014). Burnout symptom sub-types and cortisol profiles: What's burning most? *Psychoneuroendocrinology, 40*, 27-36.

Maslach, C., & Jackson, S. E. (1981). The measurement of experienced burnout. *Journal of Occupational Behaviour, 2*, 99-113.

Maslch, C., & Leiter, M. (2016a). Understanding the burnout experience: recent research and its implication for psychiatry. *World Psychiatry, 15*, 103-111.

Maslach, C. & Leiter, M. (2016b). Latent burnout profiles: A new approach to understanding the burnout experience. *Burnout Research, 3*, 89-100.

Maslach, C., Schaufeli, W. B., & Leiter, M. P. (2001). Job burnout. *Annual review of psychology, 52*, 397-422.

Mather, L., Bergström, G., Blom, V., & Svedberg, P. (2014). The covariation between burnout and sick leave due to mental disorders is explained by a shared genetic liability: A prospective Swedish Twin Study with a five-year follow-up. *Twin Research and Human Genetics, 17*, 535–544.

McEwen, B. S. (1998a). Protective and damaging effects of stress mediators. *New England journal of medicine, 338*, 171-179.

McEwen, B. S. (1998b). Stress, adaptation, and disease: Allostasis and allostatic load. *Annals of the New York Academy of Sciences, 840*, 33-44.

McEwen, B. S., & Wingfield, J. C. (2003). The concept of allostasis in biology and biomedicine. *Hormones and Behavior, 43*, 2-15.

McHugo, G. J., Caspi, Y., Kammerer, N., Mazelis, R., Jackson, E., Russell, L., . . . Kimerling, R. (2005). The assessment of trauma history in women with co-occurring substance abuse and mental disorders and a history of interpersonal violence. *The journal of behavioral health services & research, 32*, 113-127.

McKinnon, W., Weisse, C. S., Reynolds, C. P., Bowles, C. A., & Baum, A. (1989). Chronic stress, leukocyte subpopulations, and humoral response to latent viruses. *Health Psychology, 8,* 389-402.

Melamed, S., Shirom, A., Toker, S., Berliner, S., & Shapira, I. (2006). Burnout and risk of cardiovascular disease: evidence, possible causal paths, and promising research directions. *Psychological bulletin, 132,* 327.

Melamed, S., Shirom, A., Toker, S., & Shapira, I. (2006). Burnout and risk of type 2 diabetes: a prospective study of apparently healthy employed persons. *Psychosomatic Medicine, 68,* 863-869.

Middeldorp, C. M., Cath, D. C., & Boomsma, D. I. (2006). A twin-family study of the association between employment, burnout and anxious depression. *Journal of Affective Disorders, 90,* 163–169.

Miller, G., Chen, E., & Cole, S. W. (2009). Health psychology: Developing biologically plausible models linking the social world and physical health. *Annual review of psychology, 60,* 501-524.

Miller, G. E., Chen, E., & Parker, K. J. (2011). Psychological stress in childhood and susceptibility to the chronic diseases of aging: moving toward a model of behavioral and biological mechanisms. *Psychological bulletin, 137,* 959-997.

Miller, G. E., Chen, E., & Zhou, E. S. (2007). If it goes up, must it come down? Chronic stress and the hypothalamic-pituitary-adrenocortical axis in humans. *Psychological bulletin, 133,* 25-45.

Miller, G. E., Cohen, S., Pressman, S., Barkin, A., Rabin, B. S., & Treanor, J. J. (2004). Psychological stress and antibody response to influenza vaccination: when is the critical period for stress, and how does it get inside the body? *Psychosomatic Medicine, 66,* 215-223.

Miller, G. E., Cohen, S., & Ritchey, A. K. (2002). Chronic psychological stress and the regulation of pro-inflammatory cytokines: a glucocorticoid-resistance model. *Health Psychology, 21,* 531-541.

Miller, G. E., Rohleder, N., Stetler, C., & Kirschbaum, C. (2005). Clinical depression and regulation of the inflammatory response during acute stress. *Psychosomatic Medicine, 67,* 679-687.

Mommersteeg, P. M., Heijnen, C. J., Kavelaars, A., & van Doornen, L. J. (2006). Immune and endocrine function in burnout syndrome. *Psychosomatic Medicine, 68,* 879-886.

Mommersteeg, P. M., Heijnen, C. J., Verbraak, M. J., & van Doornen, L. J. (2006a). Clinical burnout is not reflected in the cortisol awakening response, the day-curve or the response to a low-dose dexamethasone suppression test. *Psychoneuroendocrinology, 31,* 216-225.

Mommersteeg, P. M., Heijnen, C. J., Verbraak, M. J., & van Doornen, L. J. (2006b). A longitudinal study on cortisol and complaint reduction in burnout. *Psychoneuroendocrinology, 31,* 793-804.

Murri, M. B., Prestia, D., Mondelli, V., Pariante, C., Patti, S., Olivieri, B., . . . Antonioli, M. (2016). The HPA axis in bipolar disorder: systematic review and meta-analysis. *Psychoneuroendocrinology, 63,* 327-342.

Nathan, C. (2006). Neutrophils and immunity: challenges and opportunities. *Nature Reviews Immunology, 6,* 173-182.

Nicolaides, N. C., Kyratzi, E., Lamprokostopoulou, A., Chrousos, G. P., & Charmandari, E. (2015). Stress, the stress system and the role of glucocorticoids. *Neuroimmunomodulation, 22,* 6-19.

Nikkheslat, N., Zunszain, P. A., Horowitz, M. A., Barbosa, I. G., Parker, J. A., Myint, A.-M., . . . Pariante, C. M. (2015). Insufficient glucocorticoid signaling and elevated inflammation in coronary heart disease patients with comorbid depression. *Brain, behavior, and immunity, 48*, 8-18.

Nitzsche, A. (2011). *German translation of the SWING-scale.* Köln: IMVR der Universität zu Köln.

Nübling, M., Stößel, U., Hasselhorn, H.-M., Michaelis, M., & Hofmann, F. (2006). Measuring psychological stress and strain at work-Evaluation of the COPSOQ Questionnaire in Germany. *GMS Psycho-Social Medicine, 3*. Retrieved from: http://www.egms.de/en/journals/psm/2006-3/psm000025.shtml

O'connor, T., O'halloran, D., & Shanahan, F. (2000). The stress response and the hypothalamic-pituitary-adrenal axis: from molecule to melancholia. *Qjm, 93*, 323-333.

Oilman, S. E., & Siegel, J. M. (1996). Traumatic events and physical health in a community sample. *Journal of Traumatic Stress, 9*, 703-720.

Oosterholt, B. G., Maes, J. H., Van der Linden, D., Verbraak, M. J., & Kompier, M. A. (2015). Burnout and cortisol: Evidence for a lower cortisol awakening response in both clinical and non-clinical burnout. *Journal of psychosomatic research, 78*, 445-451.

Oosterholt, B. G., Maes, J. H., Van der Linden, D., Verbraak, M. J., & Kompier, M. A. (2016). Getting better, but not well: A 1.5 year follow-up of cognitive performance and cortisol levels in clinical and non-Clinical burnout. *Biological psychology, 117*, 89-99.

Otte, C., Gold, S. M., Penninx, B. W., Pariante, C. M., Etkin, A., Fava, M., . . . Schatzberg, A. F. (2016). Major depressive disorder. *Nature Reviews Disease Primers, 2*, article number 16065.

Pace, T. W., Hu, F., & Miller, A. H. (2007). Cytokine-effects on glucocorticoid receptor function: relevance to glucocorticoid resistance and the pathophysiology and treatment of major depression. *Brain, behavior, and immunity, 21*, 9-19.

Pariante, C. M. (2017). Why are depressed patients inflamed? A reflection on 20 years of research on depression, glucocorticoid resistance and inflammation. *European Neuropsychopharmacology, 27*, 554-559.

Pariante, C. M., & Lightman, S. L. (2008). The HPA axis in major depression: classical theories and new developments. *Trends in neurosciences, 31*, 464-468.

Pearlin, L. I., Schieman, S., Fazio, E. M., & Meersman, S. C. (2005). Stress, Health, and the Life Course: Some Conceptual Perspectives. *Journal of health and social behavior, 46*, 205-219.

Penz, M., Stalder, T., Miller, R., Ludwig, V. M., Kanthak, M. K., & Kirschbaum, C. (2018). Hair cortisol as a biological marker for burnout symptomatology. *Psychoneuroendocrinology, 87*, 218 - 221.

Penz, M., Wekenborg, M. K., Pieper, L., Beesdo-Baum, K., Walther, A., Miller, R., Stalder, T., & Kirschbaum, C. (2018). The Dresden Burnout Study: Protocol of a prospective cohort study for the bio-psychological investigation of burnout. *International Journal of methods in psychiatric research, 27*, e1613.

Pereg, D., Gow, R., Mosseri, M., Lishner, M., Rieder, M., Van Uum, S., & Koren, G. (2011). Hair cortisol and the risk for acute myocardial infarction in adult men. *Stress, 14*, 73-81.

Perretti, M., & Ahluwalia, A. (2000). The microcirculation and inflammation: site of action for glucocorticoids. *Microcirculation, 7*, 147-161.

Pfeiler, S., Stark, K., Massberg, S., & Engelmann, B. (2017). Propagation of thrombosis by neutrophils and extracellular nucleosome networks. *haematologica, 102*, 206-213.

Picardi, A., & Abeni, D. (2001). Stressful life events and skin diseases: disentangling evidence from myth. *Psychotherapy and psychosomatics, 70*, 118-136.

Pivonello, R., De Martino, M. C., De Leo, M., Simeoli, C., & Colao, A. (2017). Cushing's disease: the burden of illness. *Endocrine, 56*, 10-18.

Porcelli, B., Pozza, A., Bizzaro, N., Fagiolini, A., Costantini, M.-C., Terzuoli, L., & Ferretti, F. (2016). Association between stressful life events and autoimmune diseases: A systematic review and meta-analysis of retrospective case–control studies. *Autoimmunity reviews, 15*, 325-334.

Rammstedt, B., & John, O. P. (2007). Measuring personality in one minute or less: A 10-item short version of the Big Five Inventory in English and German. *Journal of Research in Personality, 41*, 203-212.

Raul, J.-S., Cirimele, V., Ludes, B., & Kintz, P. (2004). Detection of physiological concentrations of cortisol and cortisone in human hair. *Clinical biochemistry, 37*, 1105-1111.

Rhen, T., & Cidlowski, J. A. (2005). Antiinflammatory action of glucocorticoids—new mechanisms for old drugs. *New England journal of medicine, 353*, 1711-1723.

Rohleder, N. (2012). Acute and chronic stress induced changes in sensitivity of peripheral inflammatory pathways to the signals of multiple stress systems – 2011 Curt Richter Award Winner. *Psychoneuroendocrinology, 37*, 307-316.

Rohleder, N. (2014). Stimulation of systemic low-grade inflammation by psychosocial stress. *Psychosomatic Medicine, 76*, 181-189.

Rohleder, N. (2018). Burnout, hair cortisol, and timing: Hyper-or hypocortisolism? *Psychoneuroendocrinology, 87*, 215-217.

Rohleder, N., Marin, T. J., Ma, R., & Miller, G. E. (2009). Biologic cost of caring for a cancer patient: dysregulation of pro-and anti-inflammatory signaling pathways. *Journal of Clinical Oncology, 27*, 2909-2915.

Romano, M., Sironi, M., Toniatti, C., Polentarutti, N., Fruscella, P., Ghezzi, P., . . . Sozzani, S. (1997). Role of IL-6 and its soluble receptor in induction of chemokines and leukocyte recruitment. *Immunity, 6*, 315-325.

Rosmond, R. (2003). Stress induced disturbances of the HPA axis: a pathway to type 2 diabetes? *Medical Science Monitor, 9*, RA35-RA39.

Russell, E., Koren, G., Rieder, M., & Van Uum, S. (2012). Hair cortisol as a biological marker of chronic stress: current status, future directions and unanswered questions. *Psychoneuroendocrinology, 37*, 589-601.

Sapolsky, R. M., Romero, L. M., & Munck, A. U. (2000). How do glucocorticoids influence stress responses? Integrating permissive, suppressive, stimulatory, and preparative actions. *Endocrine reviews, 21*, 55-89.

Sauvé, B., Koren, G., Walsh, G., Tokmakejian, S., & Van Uum, S. H. (2007). Measurement of cortisol in human hair as a biomarker of systemic exposure. *Clinical & Investigative Medicine, 30*, 183-191.

Scapini, P., & Cassatella, M. A. (2014). Social networking of human neutrophils within the immune system. *Blood, 124*, 710-719.

Schaarschmidt, U. (2006). AVEM: Ein Instrument zur interventionsbezogenen Diagnostik beruflichen Bewältigungsverhaltens. *Unter: http://www. psychotherapie. uni-wuerzburg. de/termine/dateien/Schaarschmidt180407_AVEM. pdf (Zugriff: 10. 03. 2012).*

Schaarschmidt, U., & Fischer, A. (1996). *Arbeitsbezogenes Verhaltens-und Erlebensmuster*: Swets Test Services.

Schaufeli, W. B., & Leiter, M. P. (1996). Maslach burnout inventory-general survey. *The Maslach burnout inventory-test manual, 1*, 19-26.

Schaufeli, W. B., Leiter, M. P., & Maslach, C. (2009). Burnout: 35 years of research and practice. *Career development international, 14*, 204-220.

Schonfeld, I. S., & Bianchi, R. (2015). Burnout and Depression: Two Entities or One? *Journal of clinical psychology, 72,* 22-37.

Schwarzer, R. (1993). *Measurement of perceived self-efficacy: Psychometric scales for cross-cultural research.* Berlin, Germany: Freie Universität Berlin.

Schwarzer, R., & Schulz, U. (2002). The role of stressful life events. *Comprehensive handbook of psychology, 9,* 27-49.

Scott, K. M., Koenen, K. C., Aguilar-Gaxiola, S., Alonso, J., Angermeyer, M. C., Benjet, C., . . . Florescu, S. (2013). Associations between lifetime traumatic events and subsequent chronic physical conditions: a cross-national, cross-sectional study. *PloS one, 8,* e80573.

Segerstrom, S. C., & Miller, G. E. (2004). Psychological stress and the human immune system: a meta-analytic study of 30 years of inquiry. *Psychological bulletin, 130,* 601-630.

Seidler, A., Thinschmidt, M., Deckert, S., Then, F., Hegewald, J., Nieuwenhuijsen, K., & Riedel-Heller, S. G. (2014). The role of psychosocial working conditions on burnout and its core component emotional exhaustion-a systematic review. *Journal of Occupational Medicine and Toxicology, 9,* article number 10.

Selye, H. (1936). A syndrome produced by diverse nocuous agents. *Nature, 138,* 32.

Selye, H. (1946). The general adaptation syndrome and the diseases of adaptation. *The journal of clinical endocrinology, 6,* 117-230.

Selye, H. (1950). Stress and the general adaptation syndrome. *British medical journal, 4667,* 1383-1392.

Shields, G. S., & Slavich, G. M. (2017). Lifetime stress exposure and health: A review of contemporary assessment methods and biological mechanisms. *Social and Personality Psychology Compass, 11,* e12335.

Shirom, A., & Melamed, S. (2006). A comparison of the construct validity of two burnout measures in two groups of professionals. *International Journal of Stress Management, 13,* 176-200.

Siegrist, J., Starke, D., Chandola, T., Godin, I., Marmot, M., Niedhammer, I., & Peter, R. (2004). The measurement of effort–reward imbalance at work: European comparisons. *Social science & medicine, 58,* 1483-1499.

Siegrist, J., Wege, N., Pühlhofer, F., & Wahrendorf, M. (2009). A short generic measure of work stress in the era of globalization: effort–reward imbalance. *International archives of occupational and environmental health, 82,* 1005-1013.

Skoluda, N., Dettenborn, L., Stalder, T., & Kirschbaum, C. (2012). Elevated hair cortisol concentrations in endurance athletes. *Psychoneuroendocrinology, 37,* 611-617.

Smith, J. A. (1994). Neutrophils, host defense, and inflammation: a double-edged sword. *Journal of leukocyte biology, 56,* 672-686.

Soderstrom, M., Jeding, K., Ekstedt, M., Perski, A., & Akerstedt, T. (2012). Insufficient Sleep Predicts Clinical Burnout. *Journal of Occupational Health Psychology, 17,* 175-183.

Spiga, F., Walker, J. J., Terry, J. R., & Lightman, S. L. (2014). HPA axis-rhythms. *Comprehensive Physiology, 4,* 1273-1298.

Spitzer, R. L., Kroenke, K., Williams, J. B., & Löwe, B. (2006). A brief measure for assessing generalized anxiety disorder: the GAD-7. *Archives of Internal Medicine, 166,* 1092-1097.

Stalder, T., & Kirschbaum, C. (2012). Analysis of cortisol in hair–State of the art and future directions. *Brain, behavior, and immunity, 26,* 1019-1029.

Stalder, T., Kirschbaum, C., Alexander, N., Bornstein, S. R., Gao, W., Miller, R., . . . Fischer, J. E. (2013). Cortisol in hair and the metabolic syndrome. *The Journal of Clinical Endocrinology & Metabolism, 98,* 2573-2580.

Stalder, T., Steudte-Schmiedgen, S., Alexander, N., Klucken, T., Vater, A., Wichmann, S., . . . Miller, R. (2017). Stress-related and basic determinants of hair cortisol in humans: a meta-analysis. *Psychoneuroendocrinology, 77*, 261-274.

Stalder, T., Steudte, S., Miller, R., Skoluda, N., Dettenborn, L., & Kirschbaum, C. (2012). Intraindividual stability of hair cortisol concentrations. *Psychoneuroendocrinology, 37*, 602-610.

Staufenbiel, S. M., Penninx, B. W., Spijker, A. T., Elzinga, B. M., & van Rossum, E. F. (2013). Hair cortisol, stress exposure, and mental health in humans: a systematic review. *Psychoneuroendocrinology, 38*, 1220-1235.

Steptoe, A., Hamer, M., & Chida, Y. (2007). The effects of acute psychological stress on circulating inflammatory factors in humans: a review and meta-analysis. *Brain, behavior, and immunity, 21*, 901-912.

Steptoe, A., & Kivimäki, M. (2013). Stress and cardiovascular disease: an update on current knowledge. *Annual review of public health, 34*, 337-354.

Steudte-Schmiedgen, S., Kirschbaum, C., Alexander, N., & Stalder, T. (2016). An integrative model linking traumatization, cortisol dysregulation and posttraumatic stress disorder: Insight from recent hair cortisol findings. *Neuroscience & Biobehavioral Reviews, 69*, 124-135.

Steudte-Schmiedgen, S., Stalder, T., Schönfeld, S., Wittchen, H.-U., Trautmann, S., Alexander, N., . . . Kirschbaum, C. (2015). Hair cortisol concentrations and cortisol stress reactivity predict PTSD symptom increase after trauma exposure during military deployment. *Psychoneuroendocrinology, 59*, 123-133.

Steudte-Schmiedgen, S., Wichmann, S., Stalder, T., Hilbert, K., Muehlhan, M., Lueken, U., & Beesdo-Baum, K. (2017). Hair cortisol concentrations and cortisol stress reactivity in generalized anxiety disorder, major depression and their comorbidity. *Journal of psychiatric research, 84*, 184-190.

Steudte, S., Kirschbaum, C., Gao, W., Alexander, N., Schönfeld, S., Hoyer, J., & Stalder, T. (2013). Hair cortisol as a biomarker of traumatization in healthy individuals and posttraumatic stress disorder patients. *Biological psychiatry, 74*, 639-646.

Steudte, S., Kolassa, I.-T., Stalder, T., Pfeiffer, A., Kirschbaum, C., & Elbert, T. (2011). Increased cortisol concentrations in hair of severely traumatized Ugandan individuals with PTSD. *Psychoneuroendocrinology, 36*, 1193-1200.

Steudte, S., Stalder, T., Dettenborn, L., Klumbies, E., Foley, P., Beesdo-Baum, K., & Kirschbaum, C. (2011). Decreased hair cortisol concentrations in generalised anxiety disorder. *Psychiatry research, 186*, 310-314.

Sulkava, S., Ollila, H. M., Ahola, K., Partonen, T., Viitasalo, K., Kettunen, J., . . . Lindström, J. (2013). Genome-wide scan of job-related exhaustion with three replication studies implicate a susceptibility variant at the UST gene locus. *Human molecular genetics, 22*, 3363-3372.

Sulkava, S., Ollila, H. M., Alasaari, J., Puttonen, S., Härmä, M., and Viitasalo, K. (2017). Common genetic variation near melatonin receptor 1A gene linked to job-related exhaustion in shift workers. *Sleep, 40*, 1–10.

Swider, B. W., & Zimmerman, R. D. (2010). Born to burnout: A meta-analytic path model of personality, job burnout, and work outcomes. *Journal of Vocational Behavior, 76*, 487-506.

Task Force of the European Society of Cardiology and the North American Society of Pacing and Electrophysiology (1996). Heart rate variability: standards of measurement, physiological interpretation and clinical use. *Circulation, 93*, 1043-65.

Tennant, C. (2002). Life events, stress and depression: a review of recent findings. *Australian and New Zealand Journal of Psychiatry, 36*, 173-182.

Thrall, G., Lane, D., Carroll, D., & Lip, G. Y. (2007). A systematic review of the effects of acute psychological stress and physical activity on haemorheology, coagulation, fibrinolysis and platelet reactivity: Implications for the pathogenesis of acute coronary syndromes. *Thrombosis research, 120*, 819-847.

Toker, S., Melamed, S., Berliner, S., Zeltser, D., & Shapira, I. (2012). Burnout and risk of coronary heart disease: a prospective study of 8838 employees. *Psychosomatic Medicine, 74*, 840-847.

Toker, S., Shirom, A., Shapira, I., Berliner, S., & Melamed, S. (2005). The association between burnout, depression, anxiety, and inflammation biomarkers: C-reactive protein and fibrinogen in men and women. *Journal of Occupational Health Psychology, 10*, 344-362.

Tomlinson, J. W., & Stewart, P. M. (2001). Cortisol metabolism and the role of 11β-hydroxysteroid dehydrogenase. *Best Practice & Research Clinical Endocrinology & Metabolism, 15*, 61-78.

Toppinen-Tanner, S., Ahola, K., Koskinen, A., & Väänänen, A. (2009). Burnout predicts hospitalization for mental and cardiovascular disorders: 10-year prospective results from industrial sector. *Stress and Health, 25*, 287-296.

Tsigos, C., & Chrousos, G. P. (2002). Hypothalamic–pituitary–adrenal axis, neuroendocrine factors and stress. *Journal of psychosomatic research, 53*, 865-871.

Turner, R. J., & Lloyd, D. A. (1995). Lifetime traumas and mental health: The significance of cumulative adversity. *Journal of health and social behavior, 36*, 360-376.

Ueda, Y., Kondo, M., & Kelsoe, G. (2005). Inflammation and the reciprocal production of granulocytes and lymphocytes in bone marrow. *Journal of Experimental Medicine, 201*, 1771-1780.

Ueda, Y., Yang, K., Foster, S. J., Kondo, M., & Kelsoe, G. (2004). Inflammation controls B lymphopoiesis by regulating chemokine CXCL12 expression. *Journal of Experimental Medicine, 199*, 47-58.

Van Der Klink, J. J., & Van Dijk, F. J. (2003). Dutch practice guidelines for managing adjustment disorders in occupational and primary health care. *Scandinavian journal of work, environment & health, 29*, 478-487.

von Känel, R., Bellingrath, S., & Kudielka, B. M. (2008). Association between burnout and circulating levels of pro-and anti-inflammatory cytokines in schoolteachers. *Journal of psychosomatic research, 65*, 51-59.

Vozarova, B., Weyer, C., Lindsay, R. S., Pratley, R. E., Bogardus, C., & Tataranni, P. A. (2002). High white blood cell count is associated with a worsening of insulin sensitivity and predicts the development of type 2 diabetes. *Diabetes, 51*, 455-461.

Ware Jr, J. E., & Sherbourne, C. D. (1992). The MOS 36-item short-form health survey (SF-36): I. Conceptual framework and item selection. *Medical care, 30, 473-483.*

Webster, J. I., Tonelli, L., & Sternberg, E. M. (2002). Neuroendocrine regulation of immunity. *Annual review of immunology, 20*, 125-163.

Wei, J., Sun, G., Zhao, L., Yang, X., Liu, X., Lin, D., . . . Ma, X. (2015). Analysis of hair cortisol level in first-episodic and recurrent female patients with depression compared to healthy controls. *Journal of affective disorders, 175*, 299-302.

Wennig, R. (2000). Potential problems with the interpretation of hair analysis results. *Forensic science international, 107*, 5-12.

Wester, V. L., & van Rossum, E. F. (2015). Clinical applications of cortisol measurements in hair. *European journal of endocrinology, 173*, M1-M10.

Wichmann, S., Kirschbaum, C., Böhme, C., & Petrowski, K. (2017). Cortisol stress response in post-traumatic stress disorder, panic disorder, and major depressive disorder patients. *Psychoneuroendocrinology, 83*, 135-141.

Wichmann, S., Kirschbaum, C., Lorenz, T., & Petrowski, K. (2017). Effects of the cortisol stress response on the psychotherapy outcome of panic disorder patients. *Psychoneuroendocrinology, 77*, 9-17.

Wingenfeld, K., Schulz, M., Damkroeger, A., Rose, M., & Driessen, M. (2009). Elevated diurnal salivary cortisol in nurses is associated with burnout but not with vital exhaustion. *Psychoneuroendocrinology, 34*, 1144-1151.

Wittchen, H. U., & Pfister, H. (1997). *DIA-X Interview*. Frankfurt a.M.: Swet Test Services.

Wolf, O. T. (2009). Stress and memory in humans: twelve years of progress? *Brain research, 1293*, 142-154.

Wolfe, J., Kimerling, R., Brown, P. J., Chrestman, K. R., & Levin, K. (1996). Psychometric review of the life stressor checklist-revised. *Measurement of stress, trauma, and adaptation*, 198-201.

World Health Organization (1992). *International Statistical Classification of Diseases and Related Health Problems: 10th Revision*. Geneva: WHO.

Zanstra, Y. J., Schellekens, J. M., Schaap, C., & Kooistra, L. (2006). Vagal and sympathetic activity in burnouts during a mentally demanding workday. *Psychosomatic medicine, 68*, 583-590.

Zarbock, A., Polanowska-Grabowska, R. K., & Ley, K. (2007). Platelet-neutrophil-interactions: linking hemostasis and inflammation. *Blood reviews, 21*, 99-111.

Ziegler-Heitbrock, L. (2007). The CD14+ CD16+ blood monocytes: their role in infection and inflammation. *Journal of leukocyte biology, 81*, 584-592.

www.ingramcontent.com/pod-product-compliance
Lightning Source LLC
LaVergne TN
LVHW041701190726
843493LV00007B/1896